The Practitioner's Guide to Nutrition-Focused Physical Exam of Infants, Children, and Adolescents

AN ILLUSTRATED HANDBOOK

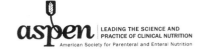

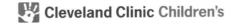

Authors

Hanna Freeman, MS, RD, CSP, LD
Pediatric Nutrition Support Team
Pediatric Institute, Cleveland Clinic Children's

Bette Klein, MS, RD, CSP, LD
Advanced Practice II Dietitian, Pediatric Nutrition Support Team
Pediatric Institute, Cleveland Clinic Children's

Sara Bewley, MS, RD, CSP, LD
Advanced Practice I Dietitian, Pediatric Nutrition Support Team
Pediatric Institute, Cleveland Clinic Children's

Merideth Miller, RD, CSP, LD
Pediatric Nutrition Support Team
Pediatric Institute, Cleveland Clinic Children's

Contributors

Jeffrey Loerch
Center for Medical Art and Photography, Cleveland Clinic

Gwen Barron, RD, CSP, LD
Pediatric Nutrition Support Team
Pediatric Institute, Cleveland Clinic Children's

Editor

Christina DeTallo, MS, MBA, RD, CSP, LD
Director, Pediatric Nutrition Support Team
Pediatric Institute, Cleveland Clinic Children's

Reviewers

Lacey Baker, MS, RD, CSP, LD, CNSC
Clinical Dietitian
Johns Hopkins All Children's Hospital, St. Petersburg, FL

Linda Heller, MS, RD, CSP, CLC, FAND
Manager of Clinical Nutrition and Lactation
Children's Hospital Los Angeles

Kristin Petrullo, DrPH(c),MPH, RD
Pediatric Medical Science Liaison
Abbott Nutrition, Columbus, OH

About ASPEN

The American Society for Parenteral and Enteral Nutrition (ASPEN) is a scientific society whose members are healthcare professionals—physicians, dietitians, nurses, pharmacists, other allied health professionals, and researchers—that envisions an environment in which every patient receives safe, efficacious, and high-quality patient care.

ASPEN's mission is to improve patient care by advancing the science and practice of clinical nutrition and metabolism.

About Cleveland Clinic Children's

Cleveland Clinic Children's is dedicated to medical, surgical, and rehabilitative care of infants, children, and adolescents. Our staff uses the latest technology and most recent research to achieve the best possible outcomes at over 40 locations across northeast Ohio. We have more than 350 pediatric specialists, who are leaders in research for cardiac care, neurological conditions, digestive diseases, and other conditions. Cleveland Clinic Children's is proud to be named a national leader in clinical care by consistently ranking among the "Best Children's Hospitals" by *U.S. News and World Report*. Our goal is to have the children and adolescents we care for back on their feet and living normal lives as quickly as possible.

https://my.clevelandclinic.org/pediatrics

Contents

Preface

The Cleveland Clinic Pediatric Nutrition Support Team (PNST) has created this illustrated nutrition-focused physical exam (NFPE) handbook to assist clinicians in performing comprehensive nutrition assessments in the pediatric population. This handbook is a resource for the identification and degree of physical depletion and malnutrition. It is imperative that the clinician understands nutrition-related concerns specific to the pediatric population because nutrition assessment is individualized to different stages of development. This handbook helps clinicians perform the NFPE on infants, children, and adolescents and addresses nutrition concerns for specialty populations, including patients with obesity, patients with neurological impairments, and patients in critical care. The NFPE is fundamental for early identification of depletion and prevention of pediatric malnutrition. For that reason, it should be a required skill set for clinicians.

Our PNST follows a systematic method during the NFPE, and we have found that a visual learning tool on how to perform the NFPE is beneficial for clinician training and standardization of methods. The photos and illustrations demonstrating exam areas and techniques in this handbook provide step-by-step guidance for the clinician and will help users build confidence in their NFPE skills.

We would like to thank the American Society for Parenteral and Enteral Nutrition (ASPEN) for giving our PNST the opportunity to collaborate on this handbook. We are grateful for our professional relationship with ASPEN and our shared core values, which include a commitment to improving patient care.

1 Introduction

The nutrition-focused physical exam (NFPE) is a critical aspect of care for pediatric patients both because the onset of malnutrition in infants and children may be rapid and because chronic malnutrition during periods of growth can delay linear maturation and impair brain function. The clinician is responsible for identifying trends indicative of faltering growth and assessing physical signs related to nutrient depletion.

The NFPE helps identify areas of muscle and fat depletion, micronutrient deficiencies, and the degree of malnutrition. Inspection and palpation are the primary exam techniques used to identify fat and muscle distribution as well as fluid shifts. Additionally, the clinician checks for alterations to the skin, nails, hair, head, and oral cavity that could be signs of micronutrient deficits or inadequate macronutrient intake. A complete NFPE helps the healthcare team understand the patient's full clinical presentation and whether nutrition intervention is warranted.

It is evident that the NFPE is an essential part of a comprehensive nutrition assessment, which will also include a thorough review of the patient's medical, surgical, and social history; anthropometrics; laboratory data; medication history; vitamin and mineral use; and dietary intake. However, although the value of an NFPE is apparent, it has not become a standard of practice—perhaps because clinicians lack sufficient training in conducting the exam and interpreting its results. This handbook is designed to be a resource for clinicians on how to complete an NFPE and identify the stages of physical depletion, vitamin and mineral deficiencies, and nutrition concerns specific to the pediatric population. Clinicians can use the techniques and tips in daily practice to gain clinical experience and enhance their skills. Additionally, this handbook provides essential information about nutrition and growth issues for specific pediatric populations: infants and toddlers; preschool- and school-age children; adolescents; children with obesity or overweight; neurologically impaired or developmentally delayed children; and critically ill patients. This targeted information helps clinicians contextualize NFPE findings for individual patients from full-term infancy through age 18 years.

▶ **TIP**

When to Perform the Nutrition-Focused Physical Exam (NFPE)

INPATIENT

The NFPE should be performed as part of the initial evaluation. Patients who are at high risk for nutritional depletion warrant a monthly full physical exam during admissions. The NFPE should be repeated with each readmission to identify significant changes that may reflect a change in nutrition status.

OUTPATIENT

The NFPE should be performed during the initial visit and during each follow-up visit if the patient is at high risk for malnutrition.

2 Nutrition Assessment

OVERVIEW

A comprehensive nutrition-focused physical exam (NFPE) is an important part of the nutrition assessment used to evaluate a patient's growth and nutrient intake. It can provide evidence that supports a diagnosis of malnutrition or another nutrition-related problem, and it helps clinicians facilitate decisions about nutrition interventions when warranted.

A complete nutrition assessment also involves the evaluation of a patient's anthropometric data (growth charts and z scores), nutrition-related medical history, laboratory data, and dietary intake. These components of pediatric nutrition assessment are briefly reviewed here. See Section 3 for information on indicators of malnutrition in pediatric patients.

ANTHROPOMETRICS

Growth assessment is the strongest indicator of nutrition status in pediatrics.

- In children younger than 24 months of age, measurements of growth include weight for age, length for age, and weight for length. *Growth velocity* is defined as the rate of change in weight or length/height over time and should be evaluated in patients from 0 to 24 months of age.[1] Any period of weight loss is likely evidence of insufficient nutrient intake to support growth.

- Head circumference is measured until 36 months of age. In young children, head circumference can be measured more accurately than length and can be used as an indicator of growth when an accurate length is not available.[2]

- In children ages 2–20 years, weight for age, height for age, and body mass index (BMI) for age are obtained. BMI is calculated as weight (kg) divided by height (m^2).

- Mid–upper arm circumference (MUAC) is used to assess malnutrition. Refer to the Section 5 of this handbook for additional information on MUAC.

- Triceps and subscapular skinfold thicknesses are used to evaluate regional and total body fat mass. Refer to the discussion of neurological impairment in Section 12 for additional information on these measures.

- Age-group-specific information about growth patterns is provided later in this handbook (Sections 9–11).

Measurement Techniques

Weight

- For accurate measurement of weight, children should have on minimal clothing. Infants must be in a dry diaper or naked.

- An infant scale should be used for children under 2 years of age.

- A bed scale or wheelchair scale should be used for children and adolescents who are unable to stand.

- Weight should be measured to the nearest gram for infants and the nearest 0.1 kg for older children and adolescents.

Recumbent Length (Birth to 2 Years of Age)

- Recumbent length is measured using an infantometer.

- The child's head should be held by a clinician or caregiver with the crown against the headboard so the external auditory meatus and the lower margin of the eye are aligned perpendicularly. Another clinician or caregiver carefully stretches the infant's legs by holding both ankles with one hand while moving the footboard to meet the infant's heels perpendicularly (Figure 2-1).

- The moveable footboard is used to measure length to the nearest 0.1 cm.[3]

Standing Height/Stature (Ages 2–20 Years)

- Standing height is measured with a stadiometer.

- The patient should stand with feet flat, together, and against the wall. Shoes should be removed before measurement. Legs should be straight, arms at the side, and shoulders level. The flat headpiece is lowered until it firmly touches the crown of head (Figure 2-2).

- Height is recorded to the nearest 0.1 cm.[4]

Figure 2-1. Recumbent length using an infantometer.

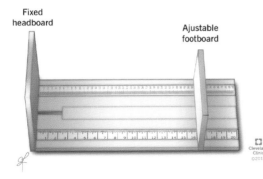

Fixed headboard

Ajustable footboard

Cleveland Clinic
©2018

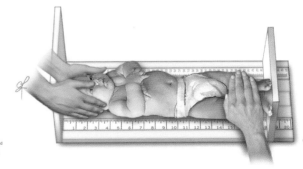

Cleveland Clinic
©2018

Figure 2-2.
Standing height measured using a stadiometer.

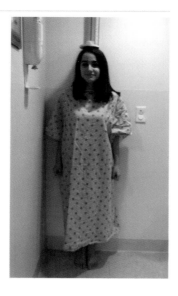

Figure 2-3. Measuring head circumference. Reprinted from Congenital zika syndrome and other birth defects. Centers for Disease Control and Prevention website. https://www.cdc.gov/pregnancy/zika/testing-follow-up/zika-syndrome-birth-defects.html. Accessed November 12, 2018.

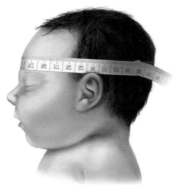

Head Circumference (Birth to Age 36 Months)

- To measure head circumference, the clinician places a nonstretchable measuring tape around the child's head so that the tape lies across the frontal bones of the skull, slightly above the eyebrows, perpendicular to the long axis of the face, above the ears, and over the occipital prominence at the back of the head (Figure 2-3). The clinician then moves the tape up and down over the back of the head to locate the maximal circumference and tightens the measuring tape so that it fits snugly around the head and compresses the hair and underlying soft tissues.

- Head circumference is measured to the nearest 0.1 cm.[5]

Mid–Upper Arm Circumference

Refer to Section 5 for discussion of how to measure MUAC.

Midparental Height

Short stature is defined as a height that plots below the 2.3rd percentile on the growth chart. Short stature can either be a variant of normal, nonpathological growth or caused by a disease. Familial (genetic) short stature and constitutional delay of growth and puberty (CDGP) are common causes of nonpathological short stature. Children with familial short stature have a normal height velocity and bone age. Individuals with CDGP have slowed linear growth velocity beginning around 3–6 months of age, in addition to delayed puberty and skeletal age. Delayed bone age causes growth to continue longer than normal, resulting in a normal adult height.[6,7]

The midparental height equation can be used to estimate a child's genetic height potential. The calculation is based on parental height and is adjusted for the sex of child (Table 2-1). If a child is growing well below their genetic height potential, referral to the appropriate specialties for further investigation is advised. Pathological causes of growth failure include undernutrition, Turner syndrome, systemic disease, growth hormone deficiency, and inflammatory bowel disease.[6,7]

Growth Charts

The 2006 World Health Organization (WHO) growth charts are recommended for use when plotting growth data for infants and children from birth to 2 years of age; these standards represent optimal growth for this age group. The WHO's 2006 Multicenter Growth Reference Study sex-specific growth standards were derived from an international sample of healthy breastfed infants and young children raised in a health-promoting environment.[8]

Growth data for children ages 2–20 years are plotted on the 2000 Centers for Disease Control and Prevention (CDC) sex-specific growth charts. The National Center for Health Statistics developed these growth charts, which are derived from data from 5 cross-sectional, nationally representative health examination surveys, in collaboration with the CDC. The CDC growth charts were most recently updated in 2000.[9]

Table 2-1. Midparental Height Equations

SEX	EQUATION
Male	[Paternal Height (cm) + Maternal Height (cm) + 13 cm]/2
Female	[Paternal Height (cm) + Maternal Height (cm) – 13 cm]/2

Table 2-2. *Z* Scores and Growth Charts for Pediatric Patients from Birth to 20 Years of Age

AGE GROUP (DATA SOURCE)	TYPES OF *Z* SCORES AND GROWTH CHARTS	RESOURCES
Birth to 2 years (World Health Organization)	• Weight for age • Length for age • Head circumference for age • Weight for length	Calculators for *z* scores and growth percentiles: https://peditools.org/growthwho Growth charts: https://www.cdc.gov/growthcharts/who_charts.htm
2–20 years (Centers for Disease Control and Prevention)	• Weight for age • Height for age • Body mass index for age	Calculators for *z* scores and growth percentiles: https://peditools.org/growthpedi Growth charts: http://www.cdc.gov/growthcharts/cdc_charts.htm

Z Scores

Z scores are the number of standard deviations above or below the mean in a normal distribution of values. They are available for weight for age, length/height for age, weight for length, head circumference for age, BMI for age, and MUAC. Compared with growth charts, z scores are preferable nutrition assessment tools because they are more descriptive than growth percentiles and quantify growth outside of percentile ranges. PediTools (www.peditools.org) provides online tools to calculate z scores if they are not available in the electronic health record.[10]

MEDICAL HISTORY

An extensive review of the patient's medical/surgical history, present illness, and clinical course can provide insight into the possible etiology of malnutrition or another nutrition-related problem.

- **Illness-related malnutrition** is associated with either an acute incident (ie, infection, burns, trauma) or a chronic medical condition (ie, congenital heart disease, inflammatory bowel disease, cystic fibrosis).

- **Non-illness-related malnutrition** can occur when behavioral, socioeconomic, and/or environmental factors result in reduced nutrient intake.[2]

LABORATORY DATA

During the nutrition assessment, the clinician should review laboratory data for indications of inflammation, micronutrient status, and fluid status. These data may confirm or rule out potential nutrition-related problems identified from the NFPE.[11]

DIETARY DATA

Food and nutrient intake has a direct effect on nutrition status. The clinician should assess intake from all sources (oral, enteral, and parenteral) and compare intake data to the individual's estimated nutrient needs in the context of his or her stage of development.[2] Nutrient intake information can be obtained from the medical record, from diet histories provided by the patient or caregiver, or by direct observation of food intake.

The Dietary Reference Intakes (DRIs) are a set of reference values used to estimate the nutrient needs of healthy individuals. The Food and Nutrition Information Center of the National Agricultural Library offers an online DRI Calculator for Healthcare Professionals (https://fnic.nal.usda.gov/fnic/dri-calculator) and publishes downloadable DRI tables (https://www.nal.usda.gov/fnic/dietary-reference-intakes).

The etiology of inadequate nutrient intake can involve factors related to acute or chronic illness, or it may be attributed to non-illness-related factors, such as starvation. The direct cause of inadequate nutrient intake can be multifactorial.

INTERVIEW TECHNIQUES AND TIPS

In the pediatric setting, a crucial step in the nutrition assessment process is to interview both the patient, if possible, and the patient's caregivers. The goals of the interview are to gather relevant information, build rapport with the patient and caregivers, and discuss the purpose of the visit. This is an opportunity to explain that the physical exam is used to evaluate baseline muscle and fat stores and look for signs of possible nutrient deficiencies.

When obtaining and sharing information, clinicians must follow the Health Insurance Portability and Accountability Act (HIPAA) guidelines to protect patient privacy.[12] The clinician must obtain consent from the patient or authorized caregiver prior to beginning the examination.

Beginning around age 3 or 4 years, children can usually answer basic questions during the interview.[13] Additionally, family and other caregivers may assist in confirming the patient's medical history and providing nutrition information needed for a comprehensive assessment. To receive additional insight pertaining to the child, the clinician should also evaluate any nonverbal cues and expressions of concern from the patient or caregiver being interviewed.

Questions about comfort level or sensitive areas should be asked before the exam begins, so the clinician can modify the exam based on the patient's needs. To the extent possible, the clinician should use layperson's terms and avoid terminology that may add to a patient's or caregiver's emotional distress. It is important to refrain from discussing any potential recovery of weight, fat, and/or muscle, as this may not be possible. In general, do not offer reassurances if they may not be achievable.

To thoroughly understand a patient's nutrition status, it is important to obtain a dietary recall and evaluate any changes in nutrient intake or behaviors. However, obtaining a complete dietary recall may be challenging if a child typically eats in a variety of settings throughout the day (daycare, school, extracurricular activities, etc).

Interview questions should probe to obtain information without leading the interviewee to a particular answer. Examples of probing interview questions related to nutrition intake include the following:

- Have you noticed a change in the amount that your child eats at meals? When did you first notice this change?

- Has the volume and/or frequency of your infant's bottle feedings changed? When did you first notice this change?

- Is your child skipping meals?

- Do your child's other caregivers express any concerns about what he/she is eating?

- Is your child receiving the prescribed infusion of enteral/parenteral nutrition or has nutrition been interrupted?

REFERENCES

1. Becker P, Carney LN, Corkins MR, et al. Consensus statement of the Academy of Nutrition and Dietetics/American Society for Parenteral and Enteral Nutrition: indicators recommended for the identification and documentation of pediatric malnutrition (undernutrition). *Nutr Clin Pract.* 2015;30(1):147–161. doi:10.1177/0884533614557642.

2. Mehta NM, Corkins MR, Lyman B, et al. Defining pediatric malnutrition: a paradigm shift toward etiology-related definitions. *JPEN J Parenter Enteral Nutr.* 2013;37:460–481. doi:10.1177/0148607113479972.

3. Beker L. Principles of growth assessment. *Pediatr Rev.* 2006;27(5):196–197.

4. Centers for Disease Control and Prevention. Measuring children's height and weight accurately at home. https://www.cdc.gov/healthyweight/assessing/bmi/childrens_bmi/measuring_children.html. Updated May 15, 2015. Accessed October 24, 2018.

5. National Health and Nutrition Examination Survey (NHANES). Anthropometry Procedures Manual. https://wwwn.cdc.gov/nchs/data/nhanes/2017-2018/manuals/2017_Anthropometry_Procedures_Manual.pdf. Updated January 2017. Accessed October 24, 2018.

6. Rogol AD. Diagnostic approach to children and adolescents with short stature. UpToDate website. https://www.uptodate.com/contents/diagnostic-approach-to-children-and-adolescents-with-short-stature?search=mid%20parental%20height&source=search_result&selectedTitle=2~20&usage_type=default&display_rank=2. Published March 2018. Accessed November 14, 2018.

7. Rogol AD. Causes of short stature. UpToDate website. https://www.uptodate.com/contents/causes-of-short-stature. Published June 2018. Accessed November 14, 2018.

8. WHO Multicentre Growth Reference Study Group. WHO child growth standards based on length/height, weight and age. *Acta Paediatr Suppl.* 2006;95:76–85. http://www.who.int/childgrowth/standards/Growth_standard.pdf. Accessed October 24, 2018.

9. Centers for Disease Control and Prevention. CDC growth charts. https://www.cdc.gov/growthcharts/background.htm. Updated August 2009. Accessed October 24, 2018.

10. PediTools. https://peditools.org. Updated February 26, 2018. Accessed April 10, 2018.

11. Green Corkins K. Nutrition-focused physical examination in pediatric patients. *Nutr Clin Pract.* 2015;30(2):203–209. doi:10.1177/0884533615572654.

12. Health Insurance Portability and Accountability Act: uses and disclosures requiring an opportunity for the individual to agree or to object. 45 CFR 164.510(b). Amended January 25, 2013.

13. Duderstadt KG, ed. *Pediatric Physical Examination: An Illustrated Handbook.* 2nd ed. St Louis, MO: Elsevier Mosby; 2014.

③ Indicators of Malnutrition

In 2015, the American Society for Parenteral and Enteral Nutrition and the Academy of Nutrition and Dietetics proposed indicators of malnutrition in pediatric patients ages 1 month through 18 years. Table 3-1 shows indicators to use on initial presentation, if only a single data point is available. Table 3-2 lists indicators for use when serial data are available from the patient's health records.

Table 3-1. Primary Indicators Recommended for the Identification and Documentation of Pediatric Malnutrition Using a Single Data Point

	MILD MALNUTRITION	MODERATE MALNUTRITION	SEVERE MALNUTRITION
Weight-for-height z score	−1 to −1.9 z score	−2 to −2.9 z score	−3 or greater z score
BMI-for-age z score	−1 to −1.9 z score	−2 to −2.9 z score	−3 or greater z score
Length-/height-for-age z score	No data	No data	−3 z score
Mid–upper arm circumference	Greater than or equal to −1 to −1.9 z score	Greater than or equal to −2 to −2.9 z score	Greater than or equal to −3 z score

BMI, body mass index.

Source: Reprinted with permission from Becker PJ, Carney LN, Corkins MR, et al. Consensus statement of the Academy of Nutrition and Dietetics/American Society for Parenteral and Enteral Nutrition: indicators recommended for the identification and documentation of pediatric malnutrition (undernutrition). *Nutr Clin Pract.* 2015;30(1):147–161. doi:10.1177/0884533614557642.

Table 3-2. Primary Indicators Recommended for the Identification and Documentation of Pediatric Malnutrition Using Serial Data

	MILD MALNUTRITION	MODERATE MALNUTRITION	SEVERE MALNUTRITION
Weight gain velocity (<2 years of age)	<75% of the norm for expected weight gain	<50% of the norm for expected weight gain	<25% of the norm for expected weight gain
Weight loss (2–20 years of age)	5% usual body weight	7.5% usual body weight	10% usual body weight
Deceleration in weight-for-length/ weight-for-height z score	Decline of 1 z score	Decline of 2 z scores	Decline of 3 z scores
Inadequate nutrient intake	51%–75% estimated energy/ protein need	26%–50% estimated energy/ protein need	≤25% estimated energy/ protein need

Source: Adapted with permission from Becker PJ, Carney LN, Corkins MR, et al. Consensus statement of the Academy of Nutrition and Dietetics/American Society for Parenteral and Enteral Nutrition: indicators recommended for the identification and documentation of pediatric malnutrition (undernutrition). *Nutr Clin Pract.* 2015;30(1):147–161. doi:10.1177/0884533614557642.

4 Overview of Physical Exam Techniques

A nutrition-focused physical examination (NFPE) of the pediatric patient uses the same techniques used for examining adults: inspection, palpation, percussion, and auscultation.[1] Inspection and palpation are the primary techniques used for the NFPE (Table 4-1).[2]

- **Inspection** includes a broad observation of aspects of the patient's physical appearance, such as the color, texture, size, smell, and symmetry of body parts.

- **Palpation** requires use of hands to examine the body by touch; it can be used to evaluate factors such as texture, temperature, muscle rigidity, and skin hydration.

Table 4-1. Exam Techniques Using Inspection and Palpation

	INSPECTION	PALPATION
Fluid	• Evaluate the overt presence and general severity of edema.	• Assess the quality and severity of edema.
Muscle and fat	• Observe the color of skin, hair, eyes, nails, and oral cavity. • Assess texture, size, and symmetry. • Inspect the contour of the abdomen.	• Examine the bulk and tone of muscle, adequacy of fat stores.
Skin	• Inspect for color, pigmentation, wounds, bruises, rashes, and textures.	• Palpate for temperature, texture, moisture, and skin turgor.
Nails	• Inspect for color, texture, and hygiene.	
Hair	• Inspect for distribution, color, texture, and pigmentation.	
Head/ orofacial areas	• **Eyes:** Inspect with a penlight for color, moisture of membranes, and any abnormalities to appearance. • **Lips:** Inspect for cracks, lesions, color, and texture. • **Mouth:** Inspect with a penlight for dental caries, baby-bottle tooth decay, teeth eruption during infancy, color, texture, swelling, lesions, and erosions.	• Palpate the top of the head on infants for the anterior fontanelle. (The anterior fontanelle usually closes around 18 months of age.[2])

CONDUCTING A SYSTEMATIC NFPE

A systematic approach to the NFPE is the most efficient method to identify muscle wasting, subcutaneous fat loss, edema, and micronutrient deficiencies. We advise newer practitioners to consistently follow these steps as they increase their clinical experience and gain confidence in their examination skills:

1. Follow facility protocols for sanitation and Contact/Isolation Precautions prior to and during the exam. Clinicians are advised to wear appropriate personal protective equipment (such as gloves and a gown) when a patient is on Contact Precautions or contact with blood or other bodily fluids is an anticipated risk.[3] To improve the accuracy and safety of the exam, gloves should not be too tight or too loose.

2. Begin with a general visual inspection of the patient.

a. Remove any external objects (blankets, clothing, gowns) that may interfere with the exam.

b. Evaluate position.

- Is the patient sitting or lying in bed?

- Proper positioning is warranted to perform an accurate exam. Identify any restrictions to positioning that may limit the clinician's ability to perform a thorough exam.

c. Evaluate body frame.

- Does the patient appear to be underweight or overweight?

- Is the patient of short stature?

- Note asymmetric features secondary to underlying medical diagnoses.

d. Assess signs of fluid status and malabsorption.

- Is there presence of edema and/or ascites?

- Does the patient appear to be dehydrated?

- Does the patient have dry, scaly skin or rashes?

3. Examine the patient from head to toe.

- Use inspection and palpation (primary techniques) as well as percussion and auscultation.

- A penlight can be used for illumination during assessment of the oral cavity and eyes.

4. Communicate with the patient or caregiver during the assessment to help identify the patient's baseline body composition status. Example questions include:

- Is your child's collarbone showing more than it used to?

- Does your child's face appear thinner to you?

- Have you [the patient or caregiver] noticed any changes in weight?

- Do your child's clothes fit looser than they used to?

- When was the last time your infant moved up to a new diaper size?

- Have you noticed any physical signs of weakness in your child?

- Have you noticed any developmental delays during infancy? (See Section 7 for information on developmental milestones.) Ask follow-up questions if delays may be related to poor nutrition status.

- Have you noticed any decline or changes in your activity level? Follow up by asking about types of activity, such as activities of daily living, school sports, gym class, and extracurricular activities (theater, choir, band, dance, etc). Identify the typical time spent during each activity and the intensity level.

- Have you seen any signs of rashes, flaking skin, or differences in hair, skin, eyes, nails, mouth, tongue, or teeth?

- Have you noticed any chewing or swallowing difficulties?

5. Review the physical exam findings in the context of findings from the clinical history and nutrition assessment (such as growth trends, weight changes, nutrient intake, functional status, and laboratory data).

REFERENCES

1. Pogatshnik C, Hamilton C. Nutrition-focused physical examination: skin, nails, hair, eyes, and oral cavity. *Support Line*. 2011;33(2):7–13.

2. Green Corkins K. Nutrition-focused physical examination in pediatric patients. *Nutr Clin Pract*. 2015;30(2):203–209. doi:10.1177/0884533615572654.

3. Centers for Disease Control and Prevention. Infection control basics. https://www.cdc.gov/infectioncontrol/basics/index.html. Updated February 2017. Accessed December 1, 2018.

5 Physical Exam of Subcutaneous Fat Loss and Muscle Wasting

OVERVIEW

The nutrition-focused physical examination (NFPE) provides valuable data for use in the diagnosis of malnutrition in children. Children are at greater risk than adults for malnutrition because children have proportionately less body fat and muscle mass than adults and higher per-kilogram energy requirements.[1-3]

In the NFPE, inspection and palpation are the primary techniques used to assess muscle and fat stores. Because it is difficult to distinguish fat loss versus muscle loss in infants and toddlers, fat and muscle stores are typically assessed together as general wasting.[1-4]

A general inspection will likely reveal obvious overweight or underweight status. In some cases, this inspection may suggest that documented anthropometric data are inaccurate and should be re-evaluated. For example, if body mass index classifies the patient as obese but weight appears normal on inspection, it could be appropriate to remeasure height and weight.

This section provides guidance in the identification of muscle and fat regions and how to classify normal status, mild to moderate depletion, and severe wasting. The NFPE is a subjective process, and clinical judgment is advised when distinguishing between mild and moderate depletion.

THE HEAD-TO-TOE APPROACH
TO REVIEWING SYSTEMS

To provide an efficient and accurate NFPE, it is imperative that the clinician understands the body's muscle and fat distribution the context of a patient's age and medical history. Figure 5-1 shows the major muscles in the body.

A head-to-toe exam provides a systematic method for an organized NFPE:

- Bony areas, hollow cheeks, and flat or baggy buttocks are signs of subcutaneous fat loss.[1]

- Protruding bone structures and hollowing of the muscle are signs of muscle wasting.[4]

A thorough, bilateral review of the body during the physical exam is important to differentiate between nutrition-related wasting and wasting from disease/deconditioned contributing factors, such as neuropathy and myopathy.

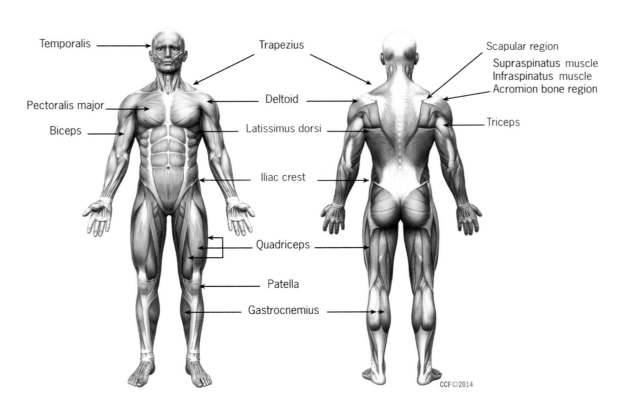

Temporalis

Trapezius

Pectoralis major

Biceps

Deltoid

Latissimus dorsi

Iliac crest

Quadriceps

Patella

Gastrocnemius

Scapular region

Supraspinatus muscle
Infraspinatus muscle
Acromion bone region

Triceps

CCF©2014

Figure 5-1. Review of major muscles in the human body.

Head and Face (Fat and Muscle)[1]

Normal

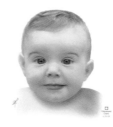 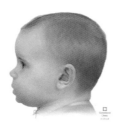 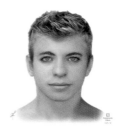 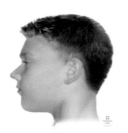

Mild to moderate malnutrition

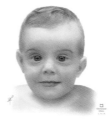 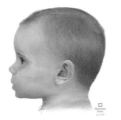 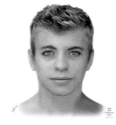 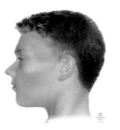

Severe malnutrition

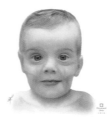 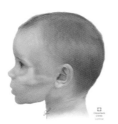 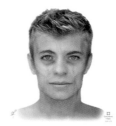 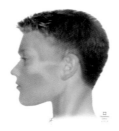

Head and Face (Fat and Muscle)[1]

	ORBITAL REGION (orbital fat pads)	BUCCAL REGION (buccal fat pads)	TEMPLE REGION (temporalis muscle)
Normal	Slightly bulging fat pads	Full, round cheeks	Well-defined muscle, flat
Mild to moderate malnutrition	Slightly dark circles, somewhat hollow	Flat cheeks, minimal bounce	Slight depression
Severe malnutrition	Dark circles, hollow appearance, loose saggy skin	Hollow, sunken cheeks	Deep hollowing/scooping

▶ EXAM TIPS

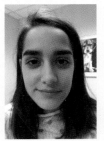

Orbital Region (orbital fat pads)

POSITIONING
Frontal view

TECHNIQUE
Lightly palpate above cheekbones.

Buccal Region (buccal fat pads)

POSITIONING
Frontal view

TECHNIQUE
Lightly palpate around buccal area.

Temple (temporalis muscle)

POSITIONING
Frontal and lateral views

TECHNIQUE
Lightly palpate temple area.

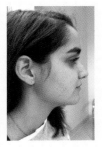

Exam Areas

Upper Body (Fat And Muscle)[1,4]

Normal

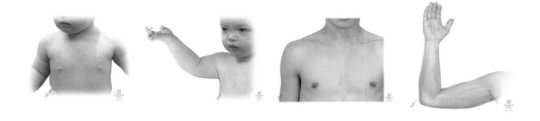

Mild to moderate malnutrition

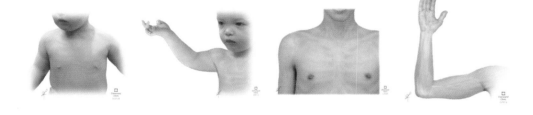

Severe malnutrition

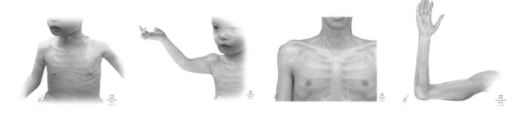

Upper Body (Fat And Muscle)[1,4]

	UPPER ARM REGION (area under the triceps muscle)	CLAVICLE BONE REGION (pectoralis major, trapezius)	ACROMION BONE REGION (deltoid muscle)
Normal	Arms full and round, ample fat tissue	Clavicle may be visible, not prominent	Rounded curves at arms, shoulders, and neck
Mild to moderate malnutrition	Some depth to pinch, not ample	Clavicle shows with some protrusion	Acromion process slightly protruded, shoulders not square
Severe malnutrition	Very little space between fingers	Clavicle protrudes and shows prominence	Shoulder-to-arm joints squared, bones prominent

▶ EXAM TIPS

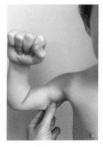

Upper Body (subcutaneous fat presence in triceps)	**Clavicle Bone Region**	**Acromion Bone Region**
POSITIONING Arm bent at 90°	**POSITIONING** As upright as possible without hunching over	**POSITIONING** Upright with arms at side
TECHNIQUE Pinch fat stores and roll between thumb and fingers to differentiate muscle and assess fat.	**TECHNIQUE** Observe line along the clavicle.	**TECHNIQUE** Observe shape from front and back.

Upper Back (Muscle)[1,4]

Normal

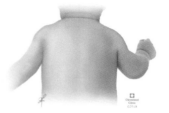
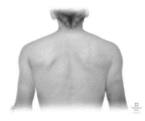

Mild to moderate malnutrition

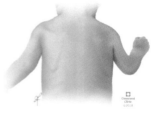
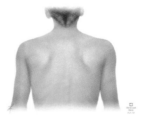

Severe malnutrition

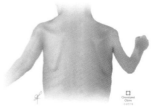
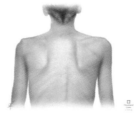

Upper Back (Muscle)[1,4]

	SCAPULAR BONE AND SPINE REGIONS (trapezius, infraspinatus, supraspinatus, latissimus dorsi, and spine)
Normal	Bone not prominent; no depressions
Mild to moderate malnutrition	Mild depression around scapula; spine or bones may show slightly
Severe malnutrition	Prominent visible scapula; spine depression is significant

▶ EXAM TIPS

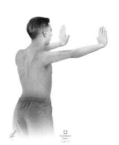

POSITIONING
Have patient push forward on object (clinician may use hand as support for patient to push against).

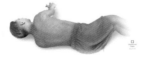

POSITIONING
If patient is unable to sit or stand, ask patient to roll to the side, extending arms as able, and push against a solid object.

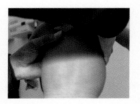

POSITIONING
For infants, have caregiver or clinician hold infant in upright position for assessment.

Exam Areas

Ribs/Midaxillary Line (Fat)[1,4]

Normal

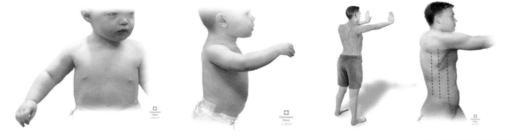

Mild to moderate malnutrition

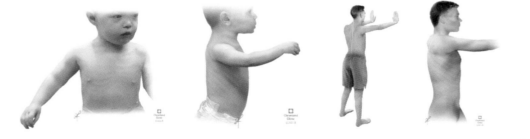

Severe malnutrition

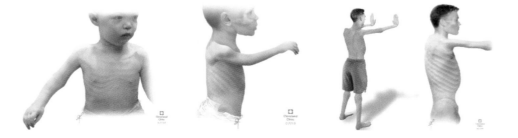

28

Ribs/Midaxillary Line (Fat)[1,4]

	THORACIC AND LUMBAR REGION (ribs, lower back, midaxillary line at iliac crest)	
Normal	• Chest is full and round with ribs not evident	• Minimal ability to visualize the iliac crest
Mild to moderate malnutrition	• Ribs are apparent with slightly visible depressions between them	• Iliac crest is slightly visible
Severe malnutrition	• Progressive prominence of ribs with loss of intercostal tissue	• Iliac crest is very visible

▶ **EXAM TIPS**

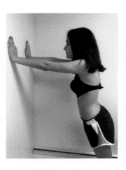

POSITIONING
Patient presses hands against solid object.

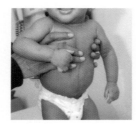

POSITIONING
For infants, have caregiver or clinician hold patient in upright position for assessment.

Lower Extremities (Muscle)[1,4]

Normal

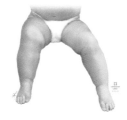 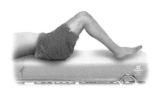 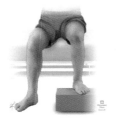

Mild to moderate malnutrition

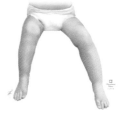 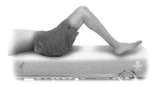 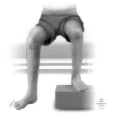

Severe malnutrition

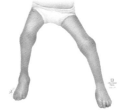 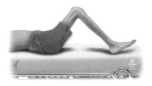 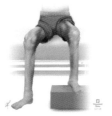

Lower Extremities (Muscle)[1,4]

	ANTERIOR THIGH REGION (quadriceps)	PATELLAR REGION (quadriceps)	POSTERIOR CALF REGION (gastrocnemius)
Normal	Well rounded, no depressions	Muscle protrudes; kneecap is not prominent	Well-developed bulb of muscle
Mild to moderate malnutrition	Slight depressions	Kneecap is more prominent	Less-developed bulb of muscle
Severe malnutrition	Significant depressions	Kneecap is prominent; little sign of muscle around knee	Thin, little to no muscle definition

▶ EXAM TIPS

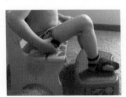

POSITIONING

Ask patient to sit up with leg propped up/ bent at the knee.

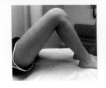

POSITIONING

If patient is unable to sit up, have patient bend knee (while lying down) so that calf and quadriceps are off the bed.

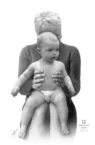

POSITIONING

For infants, have caregiver or clinician hold infant in position for assessment. An exam table can be used for assessment as needed.

TECHNIQUE

Grasp quadriceps / gastrocnemius muscle to distinguish between muscle and fat.

Lower Extremities (Fat): Limited to Infants and Toddlers[1,4]

		BUTTOCKS (gluteal fat pads)
Normal	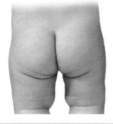	Full and round
Mild to moderate malnutrition	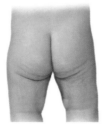	Slightly curved, but not round
Severe malnutrition	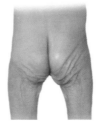	Skin is wrinkled in appearance; no fat evident

▶ **EXAM TIPS**

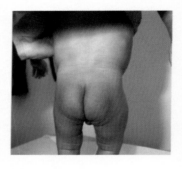

POSITIONING
Have patient stand if able.

POSITIONING
Have caregiver or clinician hold patient in position if unable to stand.

MID–UPPER ARM CIRCUMFERENCE

Mid–upper arm circumference (MUAC) should be routinely used as a tool when assessing the nutrition status of a pediatric patient.

- MUAC is a reliable measurement because this area of the body is not affected by fluid shifts caused by edema or ascites.

- Consecutive MUAC measurements can be used as a proxy for weight fluctuations when edema is present.[5]

- For patients with certain disease states, such as myopathy or genetic disorders, serial MUAC measurements may be more reflective of nutrition status than comparison to reference standards. Clinicians should always interpret measurements within the context of the patient population and clinical presentation.

- MUAC has been identified as a more sensitive prognostic indicator for mortality than weight-for-height in malnourished pediatric patients.[6]

- Z scores are available for children ages 6–59 months (World Health Organization standards) and 2 months through 18.5 years (Centers for Disease Control and Prevention standards).[7,8] The PediTools website (https://peditools.org) includes calculators for both types of z scores. See Section 3 of this handbook for guidance on interpreting MUAC z scores as indicators of malnutrition.

- Anthropometric reference data from the National Health and Nutrition Examination Survey (2011–2014) are available for patients older than 18.5 years of age.[9]

- Standardization of MUAC assessment has not yet been universally defined. Therefore, individual institutions should periodically check whether their reference standards align with current data and recommendations.

MUAC Technique

A flexible, nonstretchable measuring tape should be used to measure MUAC.

Step 1: Finding the Midpoint

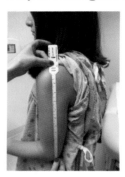

1. Bend the arm at a 90° angle with the palm facing upward.

2. Measure the arm from the posterior acromion process to the elbow (olecranon process).

3. Divide that measurement by 2 to find the midpoint. Mark this point.

Step 2: Measuring MUAC

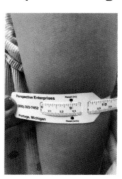

1. Relax the arm to the side of the body.

2. Wrap the flexible, nonstretchable tape around the arm at the midpoint. Use enough tape to hold it against the skin without pulling the skin. If the tape is too tight (the skin is pinched) or too loose (the tape is not touching the skin), the measurement will be inaccurate.

3. Record the measurement to the nearest 0.1 cm.

OTHER TOOLS FOR BODY COMPOSITION ASSESSMENT

In addition to MUAC, tools such as triceps skinfold thickness, bioelectrical impedance, and dual X-ray absorptiometry can be used to assess body composition.[10] These alternative methods have limitations such as expense, access to the necessary equipment, clinical status of the patient, inter-rater reliability and lack of validated reference data.[10] The clinician should review relevant data pertaining to the child's age and disease state to determine the efficacy and applicability of each tool.[10,11] (See Section 12, under "Patients with Neurological Impairments or Developmental Delays," for additional information on triceps skinfold thickness.)

REFERENCES

1. Green Corkins K, Teague EE. Pediatric nutrition assessment: anthropometrics to zinc. *Nutr Clin Pract.* 2017;32(1):40–51. doi:10.1177/0884533616679639.

2. Green Corkins K. Nutrition-focused physical examination in pediatric patients. *Nutr Clin Pract.* 2015;30(2):203–209. doi:10.1177/0884533615572654.

3. Vermilyea S, Slicker J, El-Chammas K, et al. Subjective global nutrition assessment in critically ill children. *JPEN J Parenter Enteral Nutr.* 2013;37(5):659–666. doi:10.1177/0148607112452000.

4. Secker D, Jeejeebhoy KN. How to perform Subjective Global Nutritional Assessment in children. *J Acad Nutr Diet.* 2012;112(3):424–431.e6. doi:10.1016/j.jada.2011.08.039.

5. Mehta NM, Corkins MR, Lyman B, et al. Defining pediatric malnutrition: a paradigm shift toward etiology-related definitions. *JPEN J Parenter Enteral Nutr.* 2013;37(4):460–481. doi:10.1177/0148607113479972.

6. Rasmussen J, Andersen A, Fisker AB, et al. Mid-upper-arm-circumference and mid-upper-arm circumference z score: the best predictor of mortality? *Eur J Clin Nutr.* 2012;66(9):998–1003. doi:10.1038/ejcn.2012.95.

7. World Health Organization. Arm circumference-for age. http://www.who.int/childgrowth/standards/ac_for_age/en. Accessed October 25, 2018.

8. Abdel-Rahman SM, Bi C, Thaete K. Construction of lambda, mu, sigma values for determining mid-upper arm circumference z scores in U.S. children aged 2 months through 18 years. *Nutr Clin Pract.* 2017;32 (1):68–76. doi:10.1177/0884533616676597.

9. Fryar CD, Gu Q, Ogden CL, Flegal KM. Anthropometric reference data for children and adults: United States, 2011–2014. National Center for Health Statistics. *Vital Health Stat.* 2016;3(39):1–38. https://www.cdc.gov/nchs/data/series/sr_03/sr03_039.pdf. Accessed October 25, 2018.

10. Joosten KF, Hulst JM. Nutritional assessment of the critically ill child. In: Goday, PS, Mehta NM, eds. *Pediatric Critical Care Nutrition.* New York, NY: McGraw-Hill; 2015:19–30.

11. Becker P, Carney LN, Corkins MR, et al. Consensus statement of the Academy of Nutrition and Dietetics/American Society for Parenteral and Enteral Nutrition: indicators recommended for the identification and documentation of pediatric malnutrition (undernutrition). *Nutr Clin Pract.* 2015;30(1):147–161. doi:10.1177/0884533614557642.

OVERVIEW

When completing the nutrition-focused physical exam (NFPE), it is critical to evaluate the fluid status of a patient. Dehydration, rehydration, and edema can significantly alter body weight and thus affect a patient's weight-for-length or body mass index (BMI)–for–age z scores.

Note: *Edema, which is used when assessing malnutrition in adults, is not used as an indicator of pediatric malnutrition (see Section 3 for more information about indicators used in pediatrics).*

Table 6-1. Physical Assessment for Dehydration

AREA TO EXAMINE	NORMAL	DEHYDRATED
Eyes	Membranes appear moist, and patient can produce tears.	Membranes appear dry, and patient is unable to produce tears. Eyes appear sunken.
Mouth	Saliva production is normal, and tongue is moist.	Tongue is dry and cracked.
Skin	In skin turgor test, skin returns to original position quickly.	In skin turgor test, skin returns to original position slowly.

Source: Data are from reference 1.

DEHYDRATION

In the NFPE, signs of dehydration include poor skin turgor, sunken eyes, sunken fontanel, and a dry, cracked tongue (see Table 6-1). Additionally, a lack of wet diapers and/or very dark, concentrated urine may indicate dehydration.[1,2]

- To test skin turgor, gently pinch a fold of skin between your fingers and release. The skin should return to normal/flat within 3 seconds.[1]

- Growth-velocity, weight-for-length, and BMI-for-age z score trends should not be assessed until after the patient has been rehydrated and an accurate weight has been obtained.

- Conditions that increase dehydration risks include excessive output (diarrhea or vomiting), excessive sweating, fevers, burns, increased losses via ostomies, poor oral intake, or oral intake refusal.

EDEMA

When a child has edema, it is often difficult to assess nutrition status. If edema is noted in the NFPE, it is critical to monitor fluid shifts to better assess the nutrition status of the patient. Pitting edema can be assessed by pressing an area of the skin and monitoring for remaining indentation. Refer to Table 6-2 for the 4 grades of edema.[1,3]

Table 6-2. Grading Edema

	GRADE	DEFINITION		GRADE	DEFINITION
2 mm	1+ edema	Indent ≤2 mm	6 mm	3+ edema	4–6 mm indent
4 mm	2+ edema	2–4 mm indent	8 mm	4+ edema	6–8 mm indent

Source: Data are from references 1 and 3.

REFERENCES

1. Green Corkins K. Nutrition-focused physical examination in pediatric patients. *Nutr Clin Pract.* 2015;30(2):203–209. doi:10.1177/0884533615572654.

2. Cellucci MF. Dehydration in children. Merck Manual Professional Version website. https://www.merckmanuals.com/professional/pediatrics/dehydration-and-fluid-therapy-in-children/dehydration-in-children. Accessed October 25, 2018.

3. Edema grading. Med-Health.net website. http://www.med-health.net/Edema-Grading.html. Accessed October 25, 2018.

7 Assessing Functional Status

OVERVIEW

Malnutrition can lead to decreased muscle function and strength. Malnutrition-associated loss of muscle strength is a noted predictor of postoperative complications and ability to recover from critical illness.[1] Immobility and inflammation further contribute to muscle depletion and can impair a patient's usual abilities. The malnourished child or adolescent is more likely to have frequent infections followed by a prolonged recovery, which in turn can worsen nutrition status.[1] Prolonged malnutrition can lead to developmental and cognitive delays.

MEASURING FUNCTIONAL STATUS

Handgrip Strength

Handgrip strength is highly correlated with overall muscle strength and can be used to determine functional status.[2,3] Adult studies have shown that lower handgrip strength is associated with longer hospital stays and adverse changes in nutrition status.[2] Although handgrip strength is well researched in adults, comparable data are limited for pediatric patients. Further studies are needed for complete and comparative data.

In adults and older children, a handgrip dynamometer is a simple way to measure handgrip strength (see Figure 7-1). However, measurements of handgrip strength are generally not practical in patients younger than 6 years of age; also, measuring handgrip strength requires a high degree of patient cooperation at any age.

Figure 7-1. Techniques for using a handgrip dynamometer. Reprinted with permission from reference 4: Hamilton C, ed. *Nutrition-Focused Physical Exam: An Illustrated Handbook*. Silver Spring, MD: American Society for Parenteral and Enteral Nutrition; 2016:40.

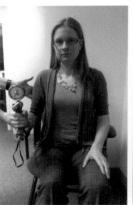
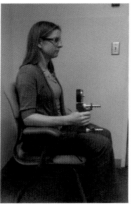
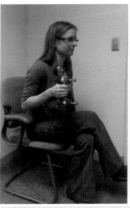
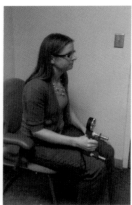

 ✔ CORRECT   ✗ INCORRECT

1. Have the patient sit upright, shoulders supported with the back of a chair; or sit on the edge of the bed, with feet touching the floor, back not hunched.

2. Testing should be performed using the dominant hand only or both hands.

3. Have the patient relax his/her arm, elbow bent at 90°.

4. The wrist should be in a neutral position.

5. Give the patient the dynamometer to hold, with their fingers wrapped around the handle (the middle finger should be at a 90° angle when gripped loosely).

6. During the test, support the patient's forearm, or support the dynamometer at the base.

7. Instruct and verbally encourage the patient to squeeze as hard as possible until the needle on the dynamometer gauge is no longer able to move. Record the result.

8. Repeat step 7 three times, then calculate the average score. Compare the result to the manufacturer's chart that accompanies the dynamometer.

Pediatric Subjective Global Nutritional Assessment

The Pediatric Subjective Global Nutritional Assessment rating form is a validated nutrition assessment tool. It includes questions about functional status that are answered by patient or parent report (see Figure 7-2). A definite loss of functional capacity is an indicator of malnutrition.[5]

Developmental Milestones

Malnutrition can affect cognitive and motor skills.[6] Decreased muscle and fat mass may make achieving developmental milestones more difficult. When assessing the patient, the clinician should note and discuss possible developmental delays or regressions with the patient's primary care physician for further assessment. For typical developmental milestones related to motor skills in infants and toddlers, refer to Table 7-1.[7]

Figure 7-2. Functional capacity section of Pediatric Subjective Global Nutritional Assessment rating form. Reprinted with permission of Elsevier from reference 5: Secker D, Jeejeebhoy KN. How to perform Subjective Global Nutritional Assessment in children. *J Acad Nutr Diet*. 2012;112(3):424–431.e6. doi:10.1016/j.jada.2011.08.039.

a) **Functional Capacity (nutritionally related):**

- ❏ no impairment, energetic, able to perform age-appropriate activity

- ❏ restricted in physically strenuous activity, but able to perform play and/or school activities in a light or sedentary nature; less energy; tired more often

- ❏ little or no play or activities, confined to bed or chair >50% of waking time; no energy; sleeps often

b) **Function in the past 2 weeks:**

- ❏ no change

- ❏ increased

- ❏ decreased

Table 7-1. Typical Motor Skill Development of Infants and Toddlers (Birth to 18 Months)

AGE, mo	DEVELOPMENTAL ACTIVITIES	AGE, mo	DEVELOPMENTAL ACTIVITIES
1–2	• When on back, kicks legs • Can hold head up for brief periods of time	9–10	• Creeps on hands and knees • Sits independently and plays with toys • May reach to play while standing at furniture • Begins to stand and walk hand-held
3–4	• Rolls from back to front • Kicks legs separately when on back • Props on forearms when on stomach • Holds head steady and erect when in supported sitting position	11–12	• Walks along furniture • May stand by self for brief periods of time • May begin walking
5–6	• Rolls from front to back • May sit with some support for short periods of time • May reach for toys when on stomach • Takes full weight on legs when held in standing position	12–18	• Walks alone • May climb stairs and run • Can push and pull toys while walking
7–8	• Plays and reaches for toys when on stomach • Rolls from stomach to back and back to stomach • Pushes up to hands and knees and may begin to rock back and forth • Sits erect when in supported sitting • May pull on furniture to stand		

Source: Data are from reference 7.

REFERENCES

1. Mehta NM, Corkins MR, Lyman B, et al. Defining pediatric malnutrition: a paradigm shift toward etiology-related definitions. *JPEN J Parenter Enteral Nutr.* 2013;37:460–481. doi:10.1177/0148607113479972.

2. Silva C, Amaral TF, Silva D, et al. Handgrip strength and nutrition status in hospitalized pediatric patients. *Nutr Clin Pract.* 2014;29(3);380–385. doi:10.1177/0884533614528985.

3. Mathiowetz V, Weimer DM, Federman SM. Grip and pinch strength norms for 6- to 19-year olds. *Am J Occup Ther.* 1986;40(10);705–711. doi:10.5014/ajot.40.10.705.

4. Hamilton C, ed. *Nutrition-Focused Physical Exam: An Illustrated Handbook.* Silver Spring, MD: American Society for Parenteral and Enteral Nutrition; 2016.

5. Secker D, Jeejeebhoy KN. How to perform Subjective Global Nutritional Assessment in children. *J Acad Nutr Diet.* 2012;112(3):424–431.e6. doi:10.1016/j.jada.2011.08.039.

6. Groce N, Challenger E, Kerac M. Stronger together: nutrition-disability links and synergies—briefing note. UNICEF website. https://www.unicef.org/disabilities/files/ Stronger-Together_Nutrition_Disability_Groce_Challenger_ Kerac.pdf. Accessed October 25, 2018.

7. Centers for Disease Control and Prevention. Developmental milestones. https://www.cdc.gov/ncbddd/actearly/ milestones/index.html. Accessed October 25, 2018.

8 Physical Exam of Hair, Eyes, Oral Cavity, Nails, and Skin

OVERVIEW

General inspection of the patient's physical appearance can help identify nutrition problems related to the intake, digestion, absorption, or metabolism of macro- or micronutrients. In particular, signs of certain macro- or micronutrient deficiencies and excesses can be recognized in the hair, eyes, oral cavity, nails, and skin.

HAIR

Inspect hair for distribution, color, and texture. Healthy hair is shiny, smooth, resilient, and not easily plucked.[1] Poor quality of hair can be associated with insufficient protein and energy intake or deficiencies of zinc, essential fatty acids, or biotin.[2]

In the newborn, all hair on the body consists of fine lanugo hair.[3] Within the first 4 months of life, an infant's hair is shed to initiate the hair growth phase.[3] Lanugo later in life can be secondary to a chronic energy deficit and subcutaneous fat depletion.[4]

Table 8-1. Nutrition-Focused Physical Assessment of Hair

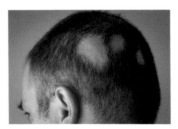

PHYSICAL SIGN	POSSIBLE NUTRIENT FINDINGS	POSSIBLE NON-NUTRIENT CAUSES
Alopecia, hair thinning, or loss	Protein, zinc, biotin, essential fatty acid, or selenium deficiency	Hypopituitarism, hypothyroidism, cancer treatment, chemical alterations, infection, psoriasis, Cushing disease, medication

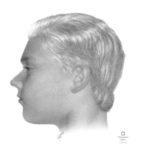

PHYSICAL SIGN	POSSIBLE NUTRIENT FINDINGS	POSSIBLE NON-NUTRIENT CAUSES
Lightened hair color	Copper, selenium, essential fatty acid, or protein deficiency	Chemical alterations

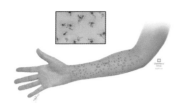

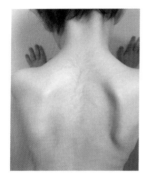

PHYSICAL SIGN
Corkscrew hair (arms, legs)

POSSIBLE NUTRIENT FINDINGS
Vitamin C deficiency

POSSIBLE NON-NUTRIENT CAUSES
Chemical alterations

PHYSICAL SIGN
Lanugo

POSSIBLE NUTRIENT FINDINGS
Energy deficiency

POSSIBLE NON-NUTRIENT CAUSES
Therapeutic steroid use, endocrine disorders

Source: Data are from references 1, 3, and 4. Photo of alopecia is from iStock.com/AlexPapp.

 ▶ **TIPS**

- Hair should be examined from above. Use of a magnified light source helps provide a sufficient view of the scalp and hair.

- Inspect scalp and hair for any lesions, dryness, or scaling.

- Palpate hair to determine whether hair is resilient and not easily plucked.

EYES

Observe eyes and conjunctivas for degree of moistness, absence or presence of swelling or lesions, and color of sclera. Healthy sclera are white.

- Examine eyes by visual inspection in a well-lit room. A penlight is useful.

- Inspect for any lesions, dryness, or swelling. Ask the patient or caregiver if the child has difficulty seeing and/or eye dryness.

- Note the color of the conjunctivas.

Table 8-2. Nutrition-Focused Physical Assessment of Eyes

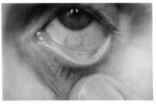

PHYSICAL SIGN	**POSSIBLE NUTRIENT FINDINGS**	**POSSIBLE NON-NUTRIENT CAUSES**
Pale conjunctiva	Anemia (iron, folate, and/or vitamin B_{12}) or copper deficiency	Low cardiac output condition

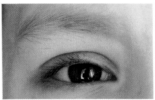

PHYSICAL SIGN	**POSSIBLE NUTRIENT FINDINGS**	**POSSIBLE NON-NUTRIENT CAUSES**
Burning, itching eyes with photophobia	Riboflavin deficiency	Allergies and eye infections

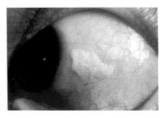

PHYSICAL SIGN	**POSSIBLE NUTRIENT FINDINGS**	**POSSIBLE NON-NUTRIENT CAUSES**
Dull, dry membrane with foamy spots	Vitamin A deficiency (Bitot's spots)	Gaucher disease

Source: Data are from reference 5. Photo of pale conjunctiva is reprinted with permission by Springer Nature from Sheth TN, Choudhry NK, Bowes M, et al. The relation of conjunctival palior to the presence of anemia. *J Gen Intern Med.* 1997;12(2):102–106. doi:10.1046/j.1525-1497.1997.00014. Photo of burning, itching eyes is by Aisylu Ahmadieva/Shutterstock.com. Photo of Bitot's spots is reprinted with permission from Baiyeroju A, Bowman R, Gilbert C, Taylor D. Managing eye health in young children. *Community Eye Health.* 2010;23(72):4–11.

ORAL CAVITY

Examination of the oral cavity can offer critical information about nutrition and hydration. The oral cavity has rapid cell turnover, usually less than 1 week.[6] The tongue should be moist and pink, with a slight rough surface with papillae.

Tooth eruption occurs between 4 and 12 months of age with the completion of primary teeth by 24 to 30 months of age. A delay in tooth eruption may be associated with severe malnutrition.[7]

Table 8-3. Nutrition-Focused Physical Assessment of the Oral Cavity

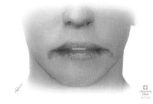

PHYSICAL SIGN	POSSIBLE NUTRIENT FINDINGS	POSSIBLE NON-NUTRIENT CAUSES
Dry, cracked, red lips	Riboflavin, niacin, or vitamin B₆ deficiency	Environmental factors, trauma

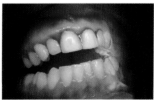

PHYSICAL SIGN	POSSIBLE NUTRIENT FINDINGS	POSSIBLE NON-NUTRIENT CAUSES
Bleeding gums	Vitamin C deficiency	Poor oral hygiene, environmental factors, trauma, hematologic conditions

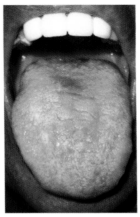

PHYSICAL SIGN
Dry mouth

POSSIBLE NUTRIENT FINDINGS
Dehydration, zinc deficiency

POSSIBLE NON-NUTRIENT CAUSES
Certain medications, cancer treatments, and systemic diseases

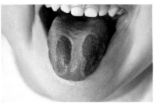

PHYSICAL SIGN
Inflamed mucosa

POSSIBLE NUTRIENT FINDINGS
Vitamin B complex, iron, or vitamin C deficiency

POSSIBLE NON-NUTRIENT CAUSES
Cancer treatments, poor oral hygiene

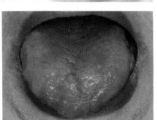

PHYSICAL SIGN
Glossitis (inflammation of tongue; red/magenta in color)

POSSIBLE NUTRIENT FINDINGS
Niacin, folate, riboflavin, iron, vitamin B_{12}, or vitamin B_6 deficiency

POSSIBLE NON-NUTRIENT CAUSES
Crohn's disease, uremia, malignancy, anticancer therapy, trauma, oral residue from recent intake of red-colored solids or fluids

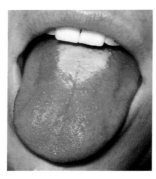

PHYSICAL SIGN
Beefy red tongue

POSSIBLE NUTRIENT FINDINGS
Niacin, folate, riboflavin, iron, or vitamin B$_{12}$ deficiency

POSSIBLE NON-NUTRIENT CAUSES
None

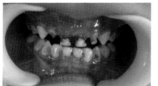

PHYSICAL SIGN
Poor dentition

POSSIBLE NUTRIENT FINDINGS
Excessive simple carbohydrate intake, bulimia

POSSIBLE NON-NUTRIENT CAUSES
Poor oral hygiene

Source: Data are from reference 5. Photo of bleeding gums is by Algirdas Gelazius/Shutterstock.com. Photo of dry mouth is reprinted from Sudarshan R, Sree Vijayabala G, Samata Y, Ravikiran A. Newer classification system for fissured tongue: an epidemiological approach. *J Tropic Med.* 2015;2015:262079. doi:10.1155/2015/262079. Photo of inflamed mucosa is by Angel Simon/Shutterstock.com. Photo of glossitis is cropped and reprinted from Kim J, Kim M-J, Kho H-S. Oral manifestations in vitamin B$_{12}$ deficiency patients with or without history of gastrectomy. *BMC Oral Health.* 2016;16:60. doi:10.1186/s12903-016-0215-y. http://creativecommons.org/licenses/by/4.0. Photo of beefy red tongue by Martin Kronawitter. https://creativecommons.org/licenses/by-sa/2.5. Photo of poor dentition reprinted with permission from Verma L, Passi S. Glass fibre-reinforced composite post and core used in decayed primary anterior teeth: a case report. *Case Rep Dentist.* 2011;2011:864254. doi:10.1155/2011/864254.

▶ TIPS

- Begin by inspecting the closed mouth for symmetry, color, or edema of the lips. Note dry, cracked lips or cracking in the corners of the mouth.

- Use a tongue depressor or gloved finger when inspecting the buccal mucosa, gums, and teeth. Normal mucosa is pinkish red, moist, and smooth. Gums should have a tight margin at each tooth and lack swelling or bleeding. It is normal for infants to display increased drooling and inflamed or swollen gums with tooth eruption.

- If the patient can follow commands, direct him or her to move tongue from side to side to help provide a complete view of the oral cavity.

NAILS

Nails should be adherent to nail bed, uniform in thickness, and smooth to touch. Nails with transverse lines may indicate protein deficiency.[9]

Table 8-4. Nutrition-Focused Physical Assessment of Nails

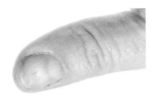

PHYSICAL SIGN	POSSIBLE NUTRIENT FINDINGS	POSSIBLE NON-NUTRIENT CAUSES
Spoon-shaped nails (koilonychia)	Iron deficiency	Trauma; hereditary or environmental factors; hematologic conditions; diabetes

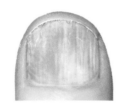

PHYSICAL SIGN	POSSIBLE NUTRIENT FINDINGS	POSSIBLE NON-NUTRIENT CAUSES
Lackluster, dull nails	Protein deficiency	Trauma, environmental factors

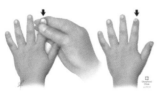

PHYSICAL SIGN	POSSIBLE NUTRIENT FINDINGS	POSSIBLE NON-NUTRIENT CAUSES
Mottled, pale nails; poor blanching	Vitamin A or C deficiency	Poor circulation

Source: Data are from references 5 and 9.

SKIN

Skin should be examined for color, texture, and temperature.

- Normal health is indicated by uniformity in skin color and skin with a soft, smooth texture, with no lesions, rashes, hyperpigmentation, or unusual temperature variation.[5]

- Abnormal skin examination findings include pallor; poor turgor; dry, scaly or flaky skin; petechiae; trauma; edema; or pressure ulcers.

Table 8-5. Nutrition-Focused Physical Assessment of Skin

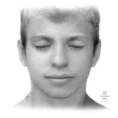

PHYSICAL SIGN	POSSIBLE NUTRIENT FINDINGS	POSSIBLE NON-NUTRIENT CAUSES
Pallor	Iron, folate, or vitamin B_{12} deficiency	Trauma, hereditary factors, diabetes, hypothyroidism

PHYSICAL SIGN	POSSIBLE NUTRIENT FINDINGS	POSSIBLE NON-NUTRIENT CAUSES
Dry, scaly skin	Vitamin A or essential fatty acid deficiency	Environmental factors, hygiene-related factors

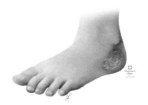

PHYSICAL SIGN	POSSIBLE NUTRIENT FINDINGS	POSSIBLE NON-NUTRIENT CAUSES
Nonhealing wounds	Zinc, vitamin C, or protein deficiency	Cellulitis, environmental factors

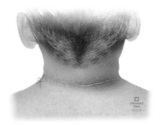

PHYSICAL SIGN
Acanthosis nigricans

POSSIBLE NUTRIENT FINDINGS
Possible indicator of insulin resistance or type 2 diabetes

POSSIBLE NON-NUTRIENT CAUSES
Hormonal disorders, medications, cancer (rare)

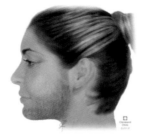

PHYSICAL SIGN
Hirsutism

POSSIBLE NUTRIENT FINDINGS
Obesity, polycystic ovary syndrome

POSSIBLE NON-NUTRIENT CAUSES
Hereditary factors

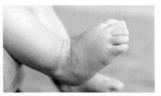

PHYSICAL SIGN
Dermatitis

POSSIBLE NUTRIENT FINDINGS
Essential fatty acid, zinc, niacin, riboflavin, or tryptophan deficiency

POSSIBLE NON-NUTRIENT CAUSES
Allergic reaction, medication, psoriasis, diaper rash

Source: Data are from references 5 and 10. Photo of dry skin is by Phanuwat Nandee/iStock.com. Photo of dermatitis is by Luca Lorenzelli/iStock.com.

 TIPS

- Use the back of your gloved hand to assess skin temperature. Skin should feel cool to the touch.

- To assess skin turgor, gently pinch a fold of skin on the back of the patient's hand or forearm between your thumb and forefinger and release. If the skin does not go back into place (remains tented), that is an indication of dehydration.

REFERENCES

1. Skin, hair, and nails. In: Ball JW, Dains JE, Flynn JA, Solomon BS, Stewart RW, eds. *Seidel's Guide to Physical Examination: An Interprofessional Approach (Mosby's Guide to Physical Examination)*. 9th ed. St. Louis, MO: Elsevier, 2019:131–183.

2. Pogatshnik C, Hamilton C. Nutrition-focused physical examination: skin, nails, hair, eye, and oral cavity. *Support Line*. 2011;33(2):7–14.

3. Duderstadt KG. *Pediatric Physical Examination: An Illustrated Handbook*. 3rd ed. St Louis, MO: Elsevier; 2014:92–94.

4. Finner AM. Nutrition and hair. *Clin Dermatol*. 2013;31(1):168–172. doi:10.1016/j.det.2012.08.015.

5. Green Corkins K. Nutrition-focused physical examination in pediatric patients. *Nutr Clin Pract*. 2015;30(2):203–209. doi:10.1177/0884533615572654.

6. Radler DR, Touger-Decker R. Nutrition screening in oral health. *Topic Clin Nutr*. 2005;20(3):181–188.

7. Sheetal A, Hiremath VK, Patil AG, Sajjansetty S, Kumar SR. Malnutrition and its oral outcome—a review. *J Clin Diagn Res*. 2013;7(1):178–180. doi:10.7860/jcdr/2012/5104.2702.

8. Xerstomia. Oral Cavity Foundation website. https://oralcancerfoundation.org/complications/xerostomia. Accessed November 15, 2018.

9. Cashman MW, Sloan SB. Nutrition and nail disease. *Clin Dermatol*. 2010;28(4):420–425. doi:10.1016/j.clindermatol.2010.03.037.

10. American Academy of Dermatology. *Acanthosis nigricans*. https://www.aad.org/public/diseases/color-problems/acanthosis-nigricans#overview. Accessed November 16, 2018.

9 Infant/Toddler Nutrition (Birth to 3 Years of Age)

OVERVIEW

During the first year of life, energy, protein, and micronutrients are primarily supplied by human milk and/or iron-fortified formula. Complementary foods are typically introduced when the infant is around the gestational age of 4–6 months. These foods should not be introduced until the infant is showing signs of developmental readiness, such as disappearance of tongue thrust, sitting with support, holding head in midline, tracking spoon with their eyes, and the ability to express the desire for solid foods.

When introduced, complementary foods that are rich in protein, zinc, and iron are recommended.[1] Foods are increased in volume and advanced in texture as the child ages and developmental skills emerge.

Fruit juice should not be introduced until the baby is at least 6 months of age. It should be 100% fruit juice and only offered from a cup to a maximum of 4 ounces per day. The clinician should assess for excessive juice intake as it can displace the nutrients provided by human milk, iron-fortified formula, and nutrient-dense foods, and also result in dental caries. Refer to Table 9-1 for selected other nutrition concerns to assess when examining infants and toddlers.

Toddlers (ages 1–3 years) continue to develop feeding skills such as chewing effectively to self-feed, using utensils, and drinking from a cup.[1] Developmental and/or motor delays may affect the child's feeding skills, which could affect the amount or types of foods consumed. In such cases, nutrition interventions may be appropriate to avoid any negative impact on nutrition status.

Toddlers may spend time with multiple caregivers throughout the day, which may make it challenging to obtain a dietary history of typical food intake. Intake at this age can be inconsistent from day to day in both volume and variety. Feeding environments can have a significant impact on the food choices and preferences of toddlers.

Table 9-1. Selected Nutrition Concerns to Assess When Examining Infants and Toddlers

POSSIBLE NUTRITION ISSUE	PHYSICAL EXAMINATION TIPS	COMMENTS
Iron deficiency anemia	• Inspect for pale-color skin (pallor), spoon-shaped nails, pale conjunctiva.	• Exclusively breastfed infants and infants who receive more than half of their daily feeds from human milk should be supplemented with 1 mg/kg/d of iron at 4 months of age until iron-containing foods are introduced.
Vitamin D deficiency (rickets)	• Inspect for bowed legs, thickening of wrists and ankles.	• Exclusively or partially breastfed infants should receive 400 IU/d of vitamin D from birth through age 12 months. • Infants consuming <1 L/d of formula should receive 400 IU/d of vitamin D.
Zinc deficiency	• Inspect for dry, flaky skin.	• Infants with chronic diarrhea are at risk for zinc deficiency.
Oral/dental problems: • Fluoride deficiency, baby-bottle tooth decay • Delayed tooth emergence during infancy	• Inspect mouth for dental caries and tooth decay. • Inspect mouth for teeth eruption during infancy.	• The clinician should assess fluoride content of water, tooth brushing status, whether infant is given a bottle while sleeping, and whether sugar or juice intake is excessive. • Delayed tooth emergence may be related to severe malnutrition.

Source: Data are from references 1–9.

GROWTH

Infants grow rapidly during the first year of life. Growth spurts generally occur at 8–12 days of life, age 3–4 weeks, and age 3 months.[1] A full-term infant's birth weight typically doubles by 5 months of age and triples by 1 year of age (see Tables 9-2 and 9-3 for classification of birth weight). Their birth length typically increases 30% by 5 months of age and increases 50% by 1 year of age.[1] Weight gain is more rapid during the first few months of life in exclusively breastfed infants and then slows in comparison to iron-fortified formula–fed infants, who may gain weight slower in the beginning and then more rapidly in later infancy.[1] Infant growth velocity (ages 0–24 months) is assessed using World Health Organization (WHO) comparative growth standards (see Section 2).

Head growth, a reflection of brain growth, is spared with prolonged undernutrition and is the last parameter to slow in velocity when an infant or toddler is malnourished.[10] Fat promotes brain development and should not be restricted in children younger than 2 years of age. Microcephaly can occur in relation to chronic malnutrition as well as genetic and disease-state factors. Head circumference trends should be evaluated in context with the weight and length trends (see Section 2). It is the clinician's responsibility to assess if there is a possible nutrition-related cause of impaired head growth.

Table 9-2. Classification of Birth Weight

CATEGORY	BIRTH WEIGHT, g
Normal birth weight	>2500
Low birth weight	1500 to <2500
Very low birth weight	1000 to <1500
Extremely low birth weight	<1000

Source: Data are from reference 1.

Table 9-3. Classification of Birth Weight for Gestational Age

CATEGORY	WEIGHT PERCENTILE
Small for gestational age	<10th
Appropriate for gestational age	10th–90th
Large for gestational age	>90th

Source: Data are from reference 1.

Note: *Prematurity, defined as less than 37 weeks' gestation, can create potential growth standard deviations.[1,11] The weight, length, head circumference, and growth trends of preterm infants should be evaluated with their degree of prematurity considered. Further discussion of prematurity is outside of the scope of this handbook.*

WHO and Centers for Disease Control and Prevention (CDC) growth charts show that growth velocity slows as children become toddlers (Table 9-4). As growth velocity slows, appetite concurrently decreases. This, coupled with the toddler's increased activity level and desire for independence, can lead to a decline in overall growth trends/percentiles. Clinicians need to assess activity level, usual intake, and eating environments that may affect growth.

Children in this age range may not be cooperative when measurements are obtained, and this may result in inaccurate data points.

Clinicians are responsible for evaluating growth trends on appropriate growth charts and should use clinical judgment if they suspect an error in measurement has occurred. Repeat measurements should be taken if necessary.

As noted in Section 2, z scores and percentiles from the CDC are used to evaluate growth in children beginning at age 2 years. The clinician should be cognizant that the percentiles from WHO and CDC do not align and that the patient should be evaluated solely on the CDC growth chart once he or she reaches 2 years of age.

Table 9-4. Average Growth Goals[a] from Birth Through Age <4 Years

AGE	WEIGHT, g/d	LENGTH, cm/mo	HEAD CIRCUMFERENCE, cm/wk
0–3 mo	28–33	3.5–3.8	0.5
3–6 mo	16–17.5	2–2.1	0.2
6–9 mo	10–11	1.5	0.1
9–12 mo	8	1.3	0.2
12–24 mo	6–7	0.9–1.0	0.2 cm/mo
2 y–<4 y	3.5–5	0.5–0.7	N/A

[a] The growth velocity goals are based on the 50th percentile for age. For ages 0–24 months, the 2006 World Health Organization growth charts are used. For ages 2 years to <4 years, growth goals are extrapolated from the 2000 Centers for Disease Control and Prevention growth charts for ages 2–20 years.

Source: Data are from references 12 and 13.

REFERENCES

1. Nevin-Folino N, ed. Infant and toddler sections. In: *Pediatric Nutrition Care Manual*. Chicago, IL: Academy of Nutrition and Dietetics; 2018.

2. American Dental Association. Statement on early childhood caries. https://www.ada.org/en/about-the-ada/ada-positions-policies-and-statements/statement-on-early-childhood-caries. Accessed October 25, 2018.

3. Cashman MW, Sloan SB. Nutrition and nail disease. *Clin Dermatol*. 2010:28(4):420–425. doi:10.1016/j.clindermatol.2010.03.037.

4. Pogatshnik C, Hamilton C. Nutrition-focused physical examination: skin, nails, hair, eye, and oral cavity. *Support Line*. 2011;33(2):7–14.

5. Green Corkins K. Nutrition-focused physical examination in pediatric patients. *Nutr Clin Pract*. 2015;30(2):203–209. doi:10.1177/0884533615572654.

6. Secker DJ, Jeejeebhoy KN. How to perform Subjective Global Nutritional Assessment in children. *J Acad Nutr Diet*. 2012;112(3):424–431.e6. doi:10.1016/j.jada.2011.08.039.

7. US National Library of Medicine. Rickets. Medline Plus website. https://medlineplus.gov/ency/article/000344.htm. Updated October 2018. Accessed October 25, 2018.

8. Baker RD, Greer FR; Committee on Nutrition American Academy of Pediatrics. Diagnosis and prevention of iron deficiency and iron-deficiency anemia in infants and young children (0-3 years of age). *Pediatrics*. 2010;126(5):1040–1050. doi:10.1542/peds.2010-2576.

9. Wagner CL, Greer FR; Section on Breastfeeding and Committee on Nutrition American Academy of Pediatrics. Prevention of rickets and vitamin d deficiency in infants, children, and adolescents. *Pediatrics*. 2008;122(5): 1142–1152. doi:10.1542/peds.2008-1862.

10. University of Texas Medical Branch. Nutrition in infancy, childhood and youth: failure to thrive. In: *Core Concepts of Pediatrics*. 2nd ed. https://www.utmb.edu/Pedi_Ed/CoreV2/Nutrition/Nutrition14.html. Accessed October 25, 2018.

11. Graber E. Physical growth of infants and children. Merck Manual Professional Version website. https://www.merckmanuals.com/professional/pediatrics/growth-and-development/physical-growth-of-infants-and-children. Accessed October 25, 2018.

12. World Health Organization. Child growth standards. www.who.int/childgrowth/standards/w_velocity/en. Accessed November 26, 2018.

13. Centers for Disease Control and Prevention. Clinical growth charts. https://www.cdc.gov/growthcharts/clinical_charts.htm. Accessed November 26, 2018.

10 Childhood Nutrition (Ages 3 to <11 Years)

OVERVIEW

Preschool-age children (ages 3–4 years) have typically mastered the oral motor skills needed to eat a variety of foods. The clinician is responsible for evaluating delays in such skills because they may affect nutrition status.

Accurate diet histories may be challenging to obtain because preschool-age children eat their meals and snacks in a variety of places throughout the day (eg, home, other residences, preschool, daycare). When meeting with the parent or primary caregiver, try to get an overall sense of eating behaviors, keeping in mind that those behaviors might be different when the child is in the presence of specific caregivers.[1]

Overall nutrition goals for school-age children (ages 5–11 years) are to establish healthy, mindful eating habits and encourage physical activity. Children in this age group should be responding to their own internal cues about hunger and fullness. This awareness will help them to maintain a healthy body status into adulthood.

School-age children typically eat lunch (and sometimes breakfast, too) at school and may eat snacks on their own. As a result, they have more independence in food choices.[1] Also, children in this age range may begin to develop body image issues. For these reasons, the clinician conducting the nutrition-focused physical exam (NFPE) or interview may wish to speak directly with the child to get a better sense of eating behaviors. Refer to Table 10-1 for examples of nutrition concerns to assess in preschoolers and school-age children.[2-5]

Table 10-1. Selected Nutrition Concerns to Assess When Examining Preschool- and School-Age Children

POSSIBLE NUTRITION ISSUE	PHYSICAL EXAMINATION TIPS	COMMENTS
Iron deficiency anemia	• Inspect for pale-color skin (pallor), spoon-shaped nails, pale conjunctiva.	• Low intake of iron-containing foods and excessive milk intake may be associated with iron deficiency anemia.
Dental caries	• Inspect mouth for tooth decay.	• Excessive sugar intake from sweetened beverages and desserts can breakdown tooth enamel.

Source: Source: Data are from references 2–5.

GROWTH

Growth velocity slows as children move from being toddlers to being preschoolers. The clinician should reassure caregivers that it is normal for appetite to decline as growth slows.

When assessing a child's body mass index (BMI), remember to look at the entire picture, including the family's heights and body frames (see Section 2 for guidance on calculating midparental height). Also, if a BMI z score does not seem consistent with NFPE findings, mid–upper arm circumference data, and previous anthropometric trends, height and weight data should be verified because school-age children may be challenging to measure.[1] If there are any concerns about the child's body image, be mindful of them when obtaining his or her weight. BMI often increases in school-age children as their bodies prepare for puberty. It is critical to monitor trends to

determine whether adipose deposit is appropriate or excessive.[1] See Table 10-2 for average growth goals for children ages 3 to <11 years.[6]

Table 10-2. Average Growth Goals, Ages 3 to <11 Years

AGE, y	WEIGHT, g/d	HEIGHT, cm/mo
2 to <4	3.5–5	0.5–0.7
4 to <7	4.5–6.5	0.5
7 to <9	5–8.5	0.4–0.5
9 to <10	6–10	0.3–0.4
10 to <11	7–11	0.3–0.5

Growth velocity goals are based on the 50th percentile for age. Growth goals are extrapolated from the 2000 Centers for Disease Control and Prevention growth charts for ages 2–20 years.

Source: Data are from reference 6.

REFERENCES

1. Nevin-Folino N, ed. *Pediatric Nutrition Care Manual*. Chicago, IL: Academy of Nutrition and Dietetics; 2018.

2. American Dental Association. Statement on early childhood caries. https://www.ada.org/en/about-the-ada/ada-positions-policies-and-statements/statement-on-early-childhood-caries. Accessed October 25, 2018.

3. Pogatshnik C, Hamilton C. Nutrition-focused physical examination: skin, nails, hair, eye, and oral cavity. *Support Line*. 2011;33(2):7–14.

4. Cashman MW, Sloan SB. Nutrition and nail disease. *Clin Dermatol*. 2010;28(4):420–425. doi:10.1016/j.clindermatol.2010.03.037.

5. Green Corkins K. Nutrition-focused physical examination in pediatric patients. *Nutr Clin Pract*. 2015;30(2):203–-209. doi:10.1177/0884533615572654.

6. Centers for Disease Control and Prevention. Clinical growth charts. https://www.cdc.gov/growthcharts/clinical_charts.htm. Accessed November 26, 2018.

11 Adolescent Nutrition (Ages 11–20 Years)

OVERVIEW

Optimal nutrition is important during this time of rapid physical growth and development. A patient's sexual maturation rating (SMR), or Tanner stage, should be taken into account when estimating nutrient needs. For a table of SMR characteristics for each stage (1–5), see reference 1.

During the nutrition assessment of an adolescent patient, potential issues to be discussed with the patient and family include changes in weight, participation in competitive sports, social concerns, medical history, food choices (eg, the patient follows a vegetarian or vegan diet), and risk for disordered eating.[2] Refer to Table 11-1 for examples of nutrition concerns to assess in adolescents.[3-6]

Table 11-1. Selected Nutrition Concerns to Assess When Examining Adolescents

POSSIBLE NUTRITION ISSUE	PHYSICAL EXAMINATION TIPS	COMMENTS
Disordered eating	• Inspect hair for dull appearance; palpate hair for thin texture and whether it is easily plucked. • Inspect teeth for poor dentition and dental caries.	• Dull, thin, and easily pluckable hair may indicate insufficient protein intake or essential fatty acid deficiency, which may be related to an eating disorder. • Tooth decay in adolescents may be a sign of bulimia.
Iron deficiency anemia	• Inspect for pale-color skin (pallor), spoon-shaped nails, and pale conjunctiva.	• Iron deficiency anemia is a risk in patients following a vegan/vegetarian diet.
Vitamin B_{12} deficiency	• Inspect eyes for pale conjunctiva.	• A vegetarian/vegan diet may increase risk for vitamin B_{12} deficiency

Source: Data are from references 3–6.

GROWTH

Girls begin their adolescent linear growth spurt at SMR 2. SMR 2 often begins between the ages of 11 and 14 years. Completion of this growth spurt is typically associated with SMR 4.[2] The adolescent linear growth spurt in boys typically begins at SMR 4, which often falls between 13 and 15 years of age.[2] See Table 11-2 for average growth goals.[2,7] Children with disordered eating patterns may reduce their full linear potential by restricting their energy and protein intake during this vital time of rapid growth.[2]

Table 11-2. Average Growth Goals During Sexual Maturation

SEX	HEIGHT, cm/y	START OF LINEAR GROWTH SPURT
Male	7.1–12.1	SMR 4
Female	8–14	SMR 2

Abbreviation: SMR, sexual maturation rating.

Average linear growth is extrapolated from the 2000 Centers for Disease Control and Prevention growth charts for ages 2–20 years.

Source: Data are from references 2 and 7.

REFERENCES

1. Annex H: Sexual maturity rating (Tanner staging) in adolescents. In: *Antiretroviral Therapy for HIV Infection in Infants and Children: Towards Universal Access: Recommendations for a Public Health Approach: 2010 Revision.* Geneva, Switzerland: World Health Organization; 2010. National Center for Biotechnology Information website. https://www.ncbi.nlm.nih.gov/books/NBK138588. Accessed October 26, 2018.

2. Nevin-Folino N, ed. *Pediatric Nutrition Care Manual.* Chicago, IL: Academy of Nutrition and Dietetics; 2018.

3. Pogatshnik C, Hamilton C. Nutrition-focused physical examination: skin, nails, hair, eye, and oral cavity. *Support Line.* 2011;33(2):7–14.

4. Cashman MW, Sloan SB. Nutrition and nail disease. *Clin Dermatol.* 2010;28(4):420–425. doi:10.1016/j.clindermatol.2010.03.037

5. Green Corkins K. Nutrition-focused physical examination in pediatric patients. *Nutr Clin Pract.* 2015;30(2):203–209. doi:10.1177/0884533615572654.

6. Secker DJ, Jeejeebhoy KN. How to perform Subjective Global Nutritional Assessment in children. *J Acad Nutr Diet.* 2012;112(3):424–431.e6. doi:10.1016/j.jada.2011.08.039.

7. Centers for Disease Control and Prevention. Clinical growth charts. https://www.cdc.gov/growthcharts/clinical_charts.htm. Accessed December 5, 2018.

Nutrition Issues in Specialty Populations

PATIENTS WITH OBESITY OR OVERWEIGHT

Overview

Pediatric overweight or obesity can be caused by excessive nutrient intake; hormonal, genetic, or malformation conditions; and/or medications. It is the clinician's responsibility to attempt to differentiate between the etiologies of overweight or obesity.

Before conducting a nutrition-focused physical exam (NFPE), it is important to document the patient's sexual maturation rating (SMR), or Tanner stage, per physician assessment because obesity can result in early onset of puberty. During puberty, there are significant accelerations in weight and linear growth that will alter body composition.[1]

Children with obesity can be diagnosed with malnutrition in relation to their clinical presentation and physical exam. Children who are obese may not readily exhibit visual signs of muscle and fat loss because excess adipose tissue limits inspection and palpation of underlying muscle mass.[2] Clinicians should use mid–upper arm circumference (MUAC) to assess muscle wasting in obese patients who have been hospitalized for a prolonged period. Clinical judgment is advised when interpreting these results. (See Section 5 for more information on MUAC.) Refer to Table 12-1 for examples of other nutrition concerns to assess in patients with obesity or overweight.

Table 12-1. Selected Concerns to Assess When Examining Patients with Obesity or Overweight

POSSIBLE NUTRITION ISSUE	PHYSICAL EXAMINATION TIPS	COMMENTS
Acanthosis nigricans	• Inspect skin at neck, armpits, and groin for areas of dark, velvety discoloration in body folds and creases. • Palpate for thickened skin.	• If the physical exam finds indicators of *Acanthosis nigricans*, a referral to a physician or licensed independent practitioner is warranted.
Polycystic ovary syndrome	• Inspect for severe acne and excess facial and body hair.	• If the physical exam finds indicators of polycystic ovary syndrome, a referral to a physician or licensed independent practitioner is warranted.
Dental caries	• Inspect mouth for tooth decay.	• Excessive sugar intake (eg, from sweetened beverages, snacks, and desserts) can breakdown tooth enamel.

Source: Data are from references 3 and 4.

Growth

The clinician should compare the child's body mass index (BMI)–for-age percentile to the weight classifications from the National Heart, Lung, and Blood Institute (NHLBI) Expert Panel on the Identification, Evaluation, and Treatment of Overweight and Obesity (Table 12-2).[5,6] Criteria from the Centers for Disease Control and Prevention are used to define extreme obesity as Class I, II, or III.[5]

Table 12-2. Classifications of Obesity/Overweight

CLASSIFICATION	BODY MASS INDEX FOR AGE
Overweight	85th–94th percentiles
Obesity • Class I Obesity • Class II Obesity • Class III Obesity	>95th percentile • 95%–120% of the 95th percentile • 120%–140% of the 95th percentile • >140% of the 95th percentile

Source: Data are from reference 5 and 6.

PATIENTS WITH NEUROLOGICAL IMPAIRMENTS OR DEVELOPMENTAL DELAYS

Overview

Neurological impairment refers to a group of disorders involving the dysfunction of the central nervous system leading to varying forms of physical and/or mental disabilities. These disabilities can range from mild to severe impairment of function. Dysfunction may be related to a metabolic, mitochondrial, or genetic disorder or trauma to the central nervous system.

The most common diagnosis in children with neurological impairment is cerebral palsy (CP).[7] CP is a group of conditions with nonprogressive symptoms related to involuntary muscle movements. Neurological dysfunction can lead to limited adiposity in children with spasticity or excess adipose tissue in children with limited mobility. In children with severe physical delay, extremities may have severe fat absence because these children tend to store fat centrally. Patients with restricted mobility may have low energy requirements. When spasticity is present, energy needs are significantly increased.[8]

Nutrient intake may be affected by neurological dysfunction in various ways. Children with decreased muscle mass may be easily fatigued when eating and may not get adequate nutrition from oral intake. Also, when food intake is limited or energy needs are decreased, micronutrient intake may be insufficient to meet the child's requirements.[9] Some children with neurological impairment may therefore benefit from gastrostomy tube feedings to prevent and/or treat malnutrition.

Growth

Neurological impairment can lead to slowed growth related to endocrine dysfunction, the neurological impairment itself, ambulation capacity, functional ability, and/or frequent illnesses.[7] Malnutrition contributes significantly to poor growth status. Weight and stature should be measured in all patients; head circumference is measured in children under the age of 3 years. When assessing anthropometric data, the clinician must be aware that measurements of height/length may not be reliable in children with contractions, scoliosis, muscle spasms, or cognitive limitations leading to poor cooperation.

Triceps skinfold, subscapular skinfold, and mid–upper arm circumference (MUAC) data may be more accurate indicators of nutrition status than weight-for-length or BMI-for-age data alone,[10] and serial measurements of skinfolds and MUAC can be used to monitor nutrition status. See Section 5 for information on how to measure and interpret MUAC. Skinfold calipers are used to measure triceps and subscapular skinfold thicknesses (see Table 12-3).[11] Specific equations have been created to calculate body composition in children with CP using triceps and subscapular skinfolds.[12]

Table 12-3. Obtaining Skinfold Measurements Using a Skinfold Caliper

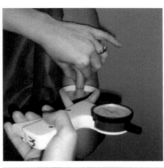

SKINFOLD
Triceps skinfold

MEASUREMENT TIPS[a]
- Measure skinfold on the posterior surface of the upper right arm, using the midpoint mark obtained for mid–upper arm circumference.
- Measurements should be repeated to verify their accuracy.

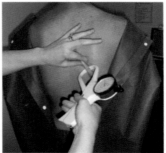

SKINFOLD
Subscapular skinfold

MEASUREMENT TIPS[a]
- Measure skinfold at the inferior angle of the right scapula.
- Measurements should be repeated to verify their accuracy.

[a] See reference 11 for full descriptions of these measurement techniques.

Source: Photos are reprinted from reference 11: Centers for Disease Control and Prevention. National Health and Nutrition Examination Survey (NHANES) Anthropometry Procedures Manual. January 2007. www.cdc.gov/nchs/data/nhanes/nhanes_07_08/manual_an.pdf. Accessed September 25, 2018.

Table 12-4. Obtaining Segmental Measurements Using an Anthropometer

BODY SEGMENT	MEASUREMENT TECHNIQUE
Upper-arm length	• Child is in a seated position or stands in an upright position, with back to the observer and arms relaxed. Elbow is flexed to 90°. • Measure the arm from the posterior acromion process to the elbow (olecranon process).
Tibial length	• Child is in a seated position, facing the clinician. • Measure from the superomedial edge of the tibia to the inferior edge of the medial malleolus.
Knee height	• Child is in recumbent position, lying on back, with knee and ankle held at 90°. • Measure height by placing the fixed blade of the caliper under the heel of the left foot and the moveable blade over the anterior surface of the thigh just behind the patella.

Source: Data are from references 13 and 14.

Segmental lengths have been studied in children with CP as alternate methods of linear measurement when patients are unable to stand or fully extend extremities for accurate measurement. Table 12-4 describes how to measure upper-arm length, tibial length, or knee height using an anthropometer.[13,14] Table 12-5 provides equations for estimating linear measurements from these segmental lengths.[14]

Table 12-5. Equations to Estimate Stature from Segmental Lengths (Ages 2–12 Years)

BODY SEGMENT	EQUATION FOR HEIGHT, cm	STANDARD ERROR
Upper-arm length (UAL)	$(4.35 \times UAL) + 21.8$	±1.7
Tibial length (TL)	$(3.26 \times TL) + 30.8$	±1.4
Knee height (KH)	$(2.69 \times KH) + 24.2$	±1.1

Source: Data are from reference 14.

Table 12-6. Growth Charts for Pediatric Patients with Neurological Impairment or Developmental Delays

DISORDER	GROWTH CHART PARAMETERS	RESOURCES
Down syndrome[a]	• Weight for age (0–36 months, 2–20 years) • Length/height for age (0–36 months, 2–20 years) • Weight for length (0–36 months) • BMI for age (2–20 years)	• Article: Zemel et al (reference 15) • Calculator for *Z* scores: PediTools (https://peditools.org/downpedi) • Growth charts: CDC (https://www.cdc.gov/ncbddd/birthdefects/downsyndrome/growth-charts.html)
Cerebral palsy[b]	• Weight for age (2–20 years) • Stature for age (2–20 years) • BMI for age (2–20 years)	• Article: Brooks et al (reference 16) • Growth charts: Life Expectancy Project (www.lifeexpectancy.org/articles/GrowthCharts.shtml)
Prader-Willi syndrome[c] (non-growth-hormone-treated)	• Weight for age (3–18 years) • Height for age (3–18 years) • Head circumference for age (3–18 years) • BMI for age (3–18 years)	• Article with growth charts: Butler et al (reference 17)
Noonan syndrome	• Weight for age (0–20 years) • Height for age (0–20 years) • BMI for age (0–20 years)	• Article with growth charts: Malaquias et al (reference 18)

Abbreviations: BMI, body mass index; CDC, Centers for Disease Control and Prevention; CP, cerebral palsy; GMFCS, Gross Motor Function Classification System; WHO, World Health Organization.

[a] Because the Down syndrome BMI charts (ages 2–20 years) describe BMI values for the sample population, they do not represent an ideal healthy distribution of BMI.[15] Use clinical judgment when interpreting these data.

[b] Separate CP-specific growth charts are available based on sex and GMFCS.[16]

[c] Use WHO growth charts for patients <2 years of age.

Diagnosis-specific growth charts are available for select patient populations known to have growth patterns unlike those of typically developing, healthy children (Table 12-6).[15-18] The Down Syndrome Growing Up Study generated sex-specific growth charts for Down syndrome infants and children from birth to 36 months and 2 to 20 years.[15] Various specialty growth charts have also been developed for patients with CP, Prader-Willi syndrome, and Noonan syndrome. Such specialty growth charts should be used with clinical judgment because the sample sizes were limited and some data are outdated. To monitor trending and proportionality, it may be useful to plot a patient's growth data on both disease-specific growth charts and the comparable WHO or CDC growth charts.[7,10,13]

PATIENTS IN CRITICAL CARE

Overview

Patients in the pediatric intensive care unit (PICU) setting are a diverse population in terms of age, disease type, interventions, comorbid conditions, and presenting nutrition status.[1] Assessment of a patient's malnutrition risk is essential in this population because malnutrition is associated with longer hospital stay; increased mortality; increased risk of hospital-acquired infections associated with venous or enteral access; and longer periods of ventilation.[19-21]

Critically ill children can become undernourished more rapidly than critically ill adults because children have proportionately less body fat and muscle mass and higher per-kilogram resting energy requirements.[22,23] Periodic nutrition reassessments are necessary to monitor for changes in nutrition status.[19] As with any patient, significant medical status changes warrant an updated NFPE.

Conducting an NFPE when a patient is in the PICU is challenging, and anthropometric data may be unreliable or unobtainable in some clinical situations (eg, trauma, burn, postoperative status, and presence of medical devices). The best practice is to obtain an accurate weight and height/length at admission; these data should be used to determine the patient's z score for BMI for age or, if the patient is younger than 2 years, the z score for weight for length. If an accurate length/height is unavailable, the patient's weight for age should be assessed.[19]

The physical examination remains an important way to evaluate muscle wasting, subcutaneous fat loss, and edema. The critically ill child often experiences third spacing in acute metabolic stress and may therefore require serial measurements to reflect change over time. Serial assessment of MUAC can be a good indicator of changes in nutrition status.

Growth

Critically ill children are at risk for nutrition deterioration during hospitalization. Periodic re-evaluation of nutrition status by the clinician is essential to modify the nutrition care plan to maintain optimum nutrition that will minimize growth failure. Body length or height is important as a point of reference for weight for length or BMI upon admission, but changes in stature are of limited value for nutrition assessment during a short-duration PICU admission.[21] Refer to Table 12-7 for additional guidance on nutrition assessment of patients in critical care or long-term care.

Table 12-7. Tips for Examining Patients in Critical Care and Long-Term Care

EXAM FOCUS	EXAM TECHNIQUE
Skin	Inspect skin for ulcers (secondary lesions), pressure injury, or nonhealing wounds. Serial evaluations are warranted.

REFERENCES

1. Rogol AD, Roemmich JN, Clark PA. Growth at puberty. *J Adolesc Health*. 2002;31(6 Suppl):192–200.

2. Secker DJ, Jeejeebhoy KN. How to perform Subjective Global Nutritional Assessment in children. *J Acad Nutr Diet*. 2012;112(3):424–431.e6. doi:10.1016/j.jada.2011.08.039.

3. Gehris RP. Dermatology. In: Zitelli BJ, McIntire SC, Nowalk AJ, eds. *Zitelli and Davis' Atlas of Pediatric Physical Diagnosis*. 7th ed. Philadelphia, PA: Elsevier; 2018:275–340.

4. Elsevier. Clinical overview: polycystic ovary syndrome. ClinicalKey website. https://www.clinicalkey.com/#!/content/clinical_overview/67-s2.0-4d576b36-0361-4939-b253-d6548de0cdac. Updated February 20, 2018. Accessed June 21, 2018.

5. Barlow SE. Expert Committee recommendations regarding the prevention, assessment, and treatment of child and adolescent overweight and obesity: summary report. *Pediatrics*. 2007;120(Suppl 4):S164–S192. doi:10.1542/peds.2007-2329C.

6. Skinner AC, Skelton JA. Prevalence and trends in obesity and severe obesity among children in the United States, 1999-2012. *JAMA Pediatr*. 2014;168(6):561–566. doi:10.1001/jamapediatrics.2014.21.

7. Kuperminc MN, Stevenson, RD. Growth and nutrition disorders in children with cerebral palsy. *Dev Disabil Res Rev*. 2008;14(2):137–146. doi:10.1002/ddrr.14.

8. American Association of Neurological Surgeons. Spasticity. http://www.aans.org/en/Patients/Neurosurgical-Conditions-and-Treatments/Spasticity. Accessed October 26, 2018.

9. Shoendorfer RB, Davies PS. Micronutrient adequacy and morbidity: paucity of information in children with cerebral palsy. *Nutr Rev*. 2010;68(12):739–748. doi:10.1111/j.1753-4887.2010.00342.x.

10. Nevin-Folino N, ed. *Pediatric Nutrition Care Manual*. Chicago, IL: Academy of Nutrition and Dietetics; 2018.

11. Centers for Disease Control and Prevention. National Health and Nutrition Examination Survey (NHANES) Anthropometry Procedures Manual. January 2007. www.cdc.gov/nchs/data/nhanes/nhanes_07_08/manual_an.pdf. Accessed September 25, 2018.

12. Gurka M, Kuperminc M, Busby M, et al. Assessment and correction of skinfold thickness equations in estimating body fat in children with cerebral palsy. *Dev Med Child Neurol*. 2010;52(2):e35–e41. doi:10.111/j.1469-8745.2009.03474.x.

13. Samson-Fang L, Bell KL. Assessment of growth and nutrition in children with cerebral palsy. *Eur J Clin Nutr*. 2013;67(Suppl 2):S5–S8. doi:10.1038/ejcn.2013.223.

14. Stevenson RD. Use of segmental measures to estimate stature in children with cerebral palsy. *Arch Pediatr Adolesc Med*. 1995;149(6):658–662.

15. Zemel BS, Pipan M, Stallings VA, et al. Growth charts for children with Down syndrome in the United States. *Pediatrics*. 2015;136(5):e1204–e1211. doi:10.1542/peds.2015-1652.

16. Brooks J, Day SM, Shavelle RM, et al. Low weight, morbidity, and mortality in children with cerebral palsy: new clinical growth charts. *Pediatrics*. 2011;128:e299–e307. doi:10.1542/peds.2010-2801.

17. Butler MG, Lee J, Manzardo AM, et al. Growth charts for non-growth hormone treated Prader-Willi syndrome. *Pediatrics*. 2015;135(1):e126-e35. doi:10.1542/peds.2014-1711.

18. Malaquias AC, Brasil AS, Pereira AC, et al. Growth standards of patients with Noonan and Noonan-like syndromes with mutations in the RAS/MAPK pathway. *Am J Med Genet A*. 2012;158A(11):2700–2706. doi:10.1002/ajmg.a.35519.

19. Mehta N, Skillman HE, Irving SY, et al. Guidelines for the provision and assessment of nutrition support therapy in the pediatric critically ill patient: Society of Critical Care Medicine and American Society for Parenteral and Enteral Nutrition. *JPEN J Parenter Enteral Nutr*. 2017;41(5):706–742. doi:10.1177/0148607117711387.

20. Goday P, Kuhn E, Sachdeva R, Mikhailov T. Does admission weight influence mortality and morbidity in the pediatric intensive care unit (PICU)? [Nutrition Week scientific abstract] *JPEN J Parenter Enteral Nutr*. 2008;32:316–317. doi:10.1177/0148-60710317921.

21. Joosten KF, Hulst JM. Nutritional assessment of the critically ill child. In: Goday PS, Mehta NM, eds. Pediatric Critical Care Nutrition. New York, NY: McGraw-Hill; 2015:19–30.

22. Mehta NM, Corkins MR, Lyman B, et al. Defining pediatric malnutrition: a paradigm shift toward etiology-related definitions. *JPEN J Parenter Enteral Nutr*. 2013;37:460–481. doi:10.1177/0148607113479972.

23. Vermilyea S, Slicker J, Chammas K, et al. Subjective Global Nutrition Assessment in critically ill children. *JPEN J Parenter Enteral Nutr*. 2013;37(5);659–666. doi:10.1177/0148607112452000.